100 Questions & Answers About Cancer Symptoms and Cancer Treatment Side Effects
Second Edition

Joanne Frankel Kelvin,
RN, MSN, AOCN
Memorial Sloan-Kettering Cancer Center

Leslie B. Tyson,
MS, APN-BC, OCN
Memorial Sloan-Kettering Cancer Center

JONES AND BARTLETT PUBLISHERS
Sudbury, Massachusetts
BOSTON   TORONTO   LONDON   SINGAPORE

616.994
KEL

World Headquarters

Jones and Bartlett
  Publishers
40 Tall Pine Drive
Sudbury, MA 01776
978-443-5000
info@jbpub.com
www.jbpub.com

Jones and Bartlett
  Publishers Canada
6339 Ormindale Way
Mississauga, Ontario L5V 1J2
Canada

Jones and Bartlett
  Publishers International
Barb House, Barb Mews
London W6 7PA
United Kingdom

Jones and Bartlett's books and products are available through most bookstores and online booksellers. To contact Jones and Bartlett Publishers directly, call 800-832-0034, fax 978-443-8000, or visit our website, www.jbpub.com.

> Substantial discounts on bulk quantities of Jones and Bartlett's publications are available to corporations, professional associations, and other qualified organizations. For details and specific discount information, contact the special sales department at Jones and Bartlett via the above contact information or send an email to specialsales@jbpub.com.

The authors, editor, and publisher have made every effort to provide accurate information. However, they are not responsible for errors, omissions, or for any outcomes related to the use of the contents of this book and take no responsibility for the use of the products and procedures described. Treatments and side effects described in this book may not be applicable to all people; likewise, some people may require a dose or experience a side effect that is not described herein. Drugs and medical devices are discussed that may have limited availability controlled by the Food and Drug Administration (FDA) for use only in a research study or clinical trial. Research, clinical practice, and government regulations often change the accepted standard in this field. When consideration is being given to use of any drug in the clinical setting, the healthcare provider or reader is responsible for determining FDA status of the drug, reading the package insert, and reviewing prescribing information for the most up-to-date recommendations on dose, precautions, and contraindications, and determining the appropriate usage for the product. This is especially important in the case of drugs that are new or seldom used.

Productions Credits
Executive Publisher: Christopher Davis
Editorial Assistant: Sara Cameron
Production Assistant: Lisa Lamenzo
Senior Marketing Manager: Barb Bartoszek
Manufacturing and Inventory Control Supervisor: Amy Bacus
Cover Design: Carolyn Downer
Cover Image: Top Left: © Elena Ray/Shutterstock, Inc.; Top Right: © Lisa F. Young/ShutterStock, Inc.; Bottom: © Andresr/ShutterStock, Inc.
Composition: Glyph International
Printing and Binding: Malloy, Inc.
Cover Printing: Malloy, Inc.

Library of Congress Cataloging-in-Publication Data
Kelvin, Joanne Frankel.
  100 questions & answers about cancer symptoms and cancer treatment side effects/ Joanne Frankel Kelvin, Leslie B. Tyson.—2nd ed.
    p. cm.
  ISBN 978-0-7637-7760-9
  1. Cancer—Popular works. 2. Cancer—Treatment—Complications—Popular works. 3. Antineoplastic agents—Side effects—Popular works. I. Tyson, Leslie B. II. Title. III. Title: One hundred questions and answers about cancer symptoms and cancer treatment side effects.
  RC263.K44 2011
  616.99'406—dc22
                              2010001542
6048

Printed in the United States of America
14 13 12 11 10   10 9 8 7 6 5 4 3 2 1

CONTENTS

- How do I go on with my life and start feeling "normal" again?
- How can I talk with my family and friends about my cancer?

Contents

Receiving a diagnosis of cancer presents numerous challenges: learning about your disease, selecting the physicians who will care for you, and making decisions about your treatment. Then come the day-to-day challenges: integrating the treatment schedule into your life, coping with the symptoms and side effects of the treatments, and finally making the transition to being a cancer survivor.

We hope that this book will provide information and support to help you in meeting these challenges. We have included information about cancer and cancer treatment, but the focus is on managing the symptoms of the disease and the side effects of treatment. Equally important is information we hope will help you and your family cope with the emotional and practical concerns that come up during this time. We are grateful to Jones and Bartlett for recognizing the need to offer a book such as this to people with cancer.

Joanne Frankel Kelvin, RN, MSN, AOCN
Leslie B. Tyson, MS, APN-BC, OCN

PART ONE

Cancer and Cancer Treatment

What is a cancer?

Why does cancer cause symptoms?

What are the treatments for cancer?

More . . .

1. What is a cancer?

Cancer is a term used to describe over a hundred different diseases with certain features in common. A cancer begins with a change in the structure and function of a cell that causes the cell to divide and multiply out of control. The cells can subsequently invade and damage surrounding tissues, and cells can break away and spread to other areas in the body. A cancer is generally named for the organ or type of cell in which it first begins to grow.

Cancers are generally classified as solid tumors and liquid tumors. *Solid tumors* begin in an organ of the body, such as the breast or lung. *Liquid tumors* begin in the bone marrow or lymphatic system, which carries fluids throughout the body. Examples are leukemia (cancer of the blood or bone marrow), lymphoma (cancer in the lymphatic system), and multiple myeloma (cancer of the plasma cells in the blood).

When you speak with your doctor or read information about your cancer, you'll find it easier if you understand the terms often used in speaking about cancer. A **tumor** is any abnormal mass or swelling in the body. Looking at a sample of the tumor cells under a microscope, a pathologist can determine whether it is a **benign** (noncancerous) tumor or a **malignant** (cancerous) tumor. The pathologist can also determine the tumor's **grade**, which is a measure of how abnormal the cells appear when examined under a microscope; in some cases, grade predicts how aggressive the cancer is. The **stage** is a measure of whether or not or how much the cancer has spread. To determine the stage, the doctor might order a variety of tests, such as blood tests, computed tomography (CT), magnetic resonance imaging (MRI), radionuclide scanning (e.g., bone

Tumor

An abnormal swelling or mass in the body.

Benign

Noncancerous.

Malignant

Cancerous.

Grade

A measure of how abnormal a cell appears when examined under a microscope; in some cases, grade predicts how aggressive the cancer is.

Stage

A measure of how extensive the cancer is, that is, how much it has spread.

scan), positron emission tomography (PET), and, in some types of cancer, samples of bone marrow.

Most types of cancer progress through four stages:

- In *Stage I*, the tumor is localized to a small area within the organ in which it started.
- In *Stage II*, the cancer has spread to the **lymph nodes** in the area. (Lymph nodes are bean-shaped structures in the lymphatic system that filter lymph fluid before it is returned to the bloodstream.)
- In *Stage III*, the tumor is **locally advanced** (i.e., a cancerous tumor has spread to surrounding structures).
- In *Stage IV*, the tumor has **metastasized** (i.e., a cancerous tumor has spread to a distant site, such as the bones, the liver, or the brain).

For most cancer types, the stages are defined by the American Joint Committee on Cancer (AJCC). To learn more about staging, go to www.cancerstaging.org.

2. Why does cancer cause symptoms?

The symptoms of a cancer depend on where it begins and how it grows. If the tumor is close to the surface of the body, you might see a lump or swelling, a change in color of the skin or mucous membranes, a sore that doesn't heal, or bleeding. If the tumor is deep within the body, you might not have symptoms until the tumor grows large enough to press on other structures, perhaps blocking a passageway and causing an obstruction. For example, a blockage of an airway in the lung can cause a cough, blockage of the intestine can cause constipation or vomiting, and blockage of the bile duct can cause jaundice.

As a tumor grows, it can cause pain by putting pressure on different parts of the body. A tumor may also cause

Lymph nodes

Bean-shaped structures in the lymphatic system that filter lymph fluid before it is returned to the bloodstream.

Locally advanced

A cancerous tumor has spread to surrounding structures.

Metastasized

A cancerous tumor has spread to a distant site, such as the bones, the liver, or the brain.

Cancer and Cancer Treatment

fluid to accumulate in the body. The abnormal buildup of fluid in the abdominal cavity is called **ascites**, which can cause swelling and pain in the belly. The abnormal buildup of fluid in the chest cavity is called **pleural effusion**, which can cause a cough and shortness of breath.

Symptoms from a cancer may not develop until the tumor has metastasized. For example, a spreading to the liver can cause abnormal blood tests, pain, and jaundice; a spreading to the bone can cause pain; and a spreading to the brain can cause confusion.

Having a cancer may also change the body's metabolism, causing symptoms such as weight loss, fever, sweats, and fatigue.

3. What are the treatments for cancer?

We can treat cancer in a number of ways:

- By surgery, to remove the tumor, sometimes with surrounding tissue and local lymph nodes. Surgery can also be done to remove part of a tumor or to relieve symptoms caused by the tumor (see Question 4).
- By *chemotherapy*, treatment with drugs that destroy cancer cells or stop them from growing (see Question 6 and 7).
- By *biologic therapy*, treatment with immune substances that destroy cancer cells or strengthen the ability of the immune system to destroy cancer cells (see Question 8).
- By *hormonal therapy*, treatment that alters specific hormone levels in the body by stopping the production of the hormone, blocking the hormone, or adding hormone, thereby slowing or stopping the growth of cancer cells (see Question 9).

Ascites

The abnormal buildup of fluid in the abdominal cavity.

Pleural effusion

The abnormal buildup of fluid in the chest cavity.

Chemotherapy

Treatment with drugs that destroy cancer cells or stop them from growing.

Biologic therapy

Treatment with immune substances that destroy cancer cells or strengthen the ability of the immune system to destroy the cancer cells.

Hormonal therapy

Treatment that alters specific hormone levels in the body by stopping the production of the hormone, blocking the hormone, or adding hormone, thereby slowing or stopping the growth of the cancer cells.

- By *radiation therapy*, the use of high-energy radiation to destroy cancer cells (see Question 5).

Surgery and radiation therapy are local treatments, directed to a particular part of the body. Chemotherapy, biologic therapy, and hormonal therapy are systemic treatments, which travel through the bloodstream to all parts of the body.

Cancer treatments are constantly evolving as doctors better understand the biology of how cancers start and grow and as they develop new ways to perform less invasive surgery and to more precisely deliver radiation therapy. For many cancers, doctors use *combined modality therapy*, that is, a combination of treatments.

Oncologists, doctors who specialize in the treatment of cancer, can recommend the type of treatment that is best for you. The treatment depends on the type of cancer, the stage of disease, and your general state of health. Depending on your situation, the goal of the treatment may be to cure the disease, to control the growth of the cancer, or to relieve symptoms and improve quality of life (i.e., **palliation**).

4. When is surgery used to treat cancer?

For many cancers, surgery is performed to remove the primary tumor. The local lymph nodes are often also removed for testing to determine whether the cancer has spread to the lymph nodes. If the tumor has invaded surrounding structures, they may be removed at the same time.

For some patients with locally advanced disease, radiation therapy and/or chemotherapy are given before the surgery to shrink the tumor. This increases the chance

Radiation therapy
The use of high-energy radiation to destroy cancer cells; also called radiotherapy.

For many cancers, doctors use combined modality therapy, *that is, a combination of treatments.*

Palliation
Treatment to relieve symptoms and to improve quality of life.

Cancer and Cancer Treatment

that the entire tumor can be resected or removed. In some cases, it also allows for resection of the tumor without the need to remove surrounding structures. For example, this approach may be used with a cancer in the rectum, to avoid having to also remove the anus and create a permanent colostomy or opening in the skin for defecation.

Surgery can also be done to resect part of a tumor or to relieve symptoms that a tumor causes. Examples are surgery to remove a metastatic tumor in the brain, to bypass a blockage of the intestine, or to repair a bone broken from the spread of the cancer.

5. What is radiation therapy, and how is it given?

Radiation therapy treats disease with high-energy waves or particles. Radiation therapy is most commonly administered as external beam treatment. Beams of radiation are directed from a machine outside the body, such as a linear accelerator, to the affected part of the body. As the energy passes through the body, it damages the cells in its path. Cancer cells are destroyed, obliterating or shrinking the tumor. Normal cells in the path of the energy are also affected, but they are better able to recover from the radiation than cancer cells. Radiation therapy is carefully planned to deliver an accurate dose to the tumor site while minimizing the dose to the surrounding normal tissues.

Radiation therapy is carefully planned to ensure that an accurate dose is delivered to the tumor site while minimizing the dose received by the surrounding normal tissues.

Before the actual radiation treatment, you will undergo a simulation. During the simulation, you are positioned on a table, just as you will be on each day of treatment. Licensed radiation therapists may make special immobilizing devices for you, such as face masks, molds, or cradles. They will also make skin markings, usually in the form of permanent tattoos the size of a pinhead. These devices and skin markings are used to position you correctly each day of treatment. While you are in the treatment position, radiologic images are taken to localize the area to be treated. Depending on the treatment planned, the images may be taken via X-rays, CTs, MRIs, and/or PETs.

After the simulation, the radiation oncologist (the doctor who prescribes radiation therapy), working with a physicist and dosimetrist (someone who calculates amounts of radiation), develops a treatment plan. This includes the dose of radiation to give, the number of radiation beams needed, at what angles they should be directed, and how they should be shaped.

Once the planning is completed, treatment begins. Treatment does not usually require hospitalization. It is given every day, Monday through Friday, until the total dose has been delivered—generally anywhere from 2 to 9 weeks. You are usually in the treatment room for 15 to 30 minutes each day. Radiation therapists set you up in the correct position and then leave the room. Using controls outside the room, they turn on the radiation beam, which stays on for about 5 to 15 minutes. When the beam is on, you feel nothing; there is no pain, burning, or discomfort. You may see the treatment machine move around you to the different positions needed to deliver each beam, and you hear the machine as it turns on and off.

During treatment with external beam radiation therapy, your radiation oncologist and radiation oncology nurse see you weekly. They will evaluate how you are tolerating the treatment and help you manage any side effects you develop.

We have made many advances in radiation therapy in recent years. Technological advances in planning and delivering treatment are designed to direct the radiation beams more precisely, thereby reducing the doses received by the surrounding normal tissues. You might hear your doctor mention "three-dimensional conformal radiation therapy," "intensity-modulated radiation therapy," "image-guided radiation therapy," or "stereotactic brain or body radiosurgery/radiotherapy." New machines have also been developed to deliver treatment, for example, the TomoTherapy and CyberKnife systems and machines that deliver proton therapy.

Also, treatment schedules may vary. For instance, you may receive decreased doses given more than once a day or increased doses given in only one to five treatments. In addition, chemotherapy may be given with your radiation to enhance your response to treatment.

Radiation therapy can also be administered by placing a radioactive source inside the body—an approach called internal radiation. One form of internal radiation is **brachytherapy**, radiation treatment that involves placing sealed radioactive sources (for example, seeds, wires, ribbons, or tubes) into the body. These emit radiation into the immediately surrounding area as they decay (or break down). Depending on the type of source used, it may be kept in place for 15–20 minutes or for several days. Some sources are left in place permanently and are referred to as *permanent seed implants*; these implants decay and lose their energy over time, usually a number of months.

Another form of internal radiation can be taken by mouth or injected into a vein (*radiopharmaceutical therapy*). This radioactive material travels through the

Brachytherapy

Radiation treatment that involves the placement of sealed radioactive sources (for example, seeds, wires, ribbons, or tubes) into the body that emit radiation into the immediately surrounding area as they decay (or break down); also called implant or internal radiation.

body and collects where tumor cells are located, emitting radiation until the body eliminates it.

Internal radiation may require hospitalization, and you might have to be isolated for a period of time because of the radiation your body is emitting. Your radiation oncologist and a physicist from the radiation safety service will advise you on the precautions you need to take.

Here are some sources of information on radiation therapy:

- *Radiation Therapy and You: A Guide to Self-Help During Cancer Treatment*, published by the National Cancer Institute: www.cancer.gov or 800-4-CANCER
- *American Society for Therapeutic Radiology and Oncology:* www.rtanswers.org
- *American College of Radiology:* www.radiologyinfo.org

6. What is chemotherapy, and how is it given?

Chemotherapy is the treatment of cancer with drugs. Unlike surgery and radiotherapy, which are aimed at removing or killing cancers in localized parts of the body, chemotherapy is a systemic treatment. Chemotherapy travels throughout the body and can kill cancer cells anywhere in the body. Besides destroying cancer cells, chemotherapy can damage normal, healthy cells, especially healthy cells in the lining of the mouth and gastrointestinal tract, the bone marrow, and the hair follicles. Damage to healthy cells is why chemotherapy causes side effects (see Question 13). Healthy cells can usually repair themselves, and most side effects resolve after treatment.

There are more than 100 different types of cancer, and many different chemotherapy drugs are available.

There are more than 100 different types of cancer, and many different chemotherapy drugs are available.

Your doctor will decide which chemotherapy drug(s) are right for you based on where your cancer started, on whether it has spread to other areas of your body, and on how healthy you are. For many types of cancer, your doctor will use a combination of drugs.

Chemotherapy can be given to cure the cancer, to control the disease, or to relieve symptoms (palliation). **Neoadjuvant chemotherapy** is chemotherapy treatment given before the primary treatment (such as surgery); it is used to shrink the tumor, making it easier for the surgeon to remove. Chemotherapy may also be given in this way before radiation therapy. **Adjuvant chemotherapy** is chemotherapy treatment used after a tumor has been removed surgically to destroy any microscopic cancer cells (those that cannot be seen with the naked eye) that may be left behind. For people with metastatic cancer, which usually cannot be cured, chemotherapy is the primary treatment, given to extend life and relieve symptoms.

Chemotherapy can be given in any form that other drugs are given, but it is most commonly given *intravenously* (IV), that is, through a thin needle inserted into a vein (the needle is taken out after the treatment is completed). Sometimes a special thin, flexible catheter is placed in a large vein in your body and left in place over a number of months or years, until it is no longer needed. The catheter is used for drawing blood and giving you chemotherapy, avoiding the need to stick a vein in your hand or arm. (See Question 10 for more information about catheters.) Intravenous chemotherapy can be given over minutes ("IV push"), dripped in over a number of hours, or even infused continuously over a number of days. For some types of cancer, chemotherapy is given into an artery rather

Neoadjuvant chemotherapy

Chemotherapy treatment given before the primary treatment (such as surgery) that is often used to shrink the tumor, making it easier for the surgeon to remove.

Adjuvant chemotherapy

Chemotherapy treatment and/or radiation therapy used after a tumor has been removed surgically to destroy any remaining microscopic cancer cells (those that cannot be seen with the naked eye) that may be left behind.

than a vein. (Arteries carry blood away from the heart; veins carry blood to the heart.)

Chemotherapy can also be injected under the skin (*subcutaneously*), into the muscle, or into the cerebrospinal fluid. For some types of cancer, it is infused into a body cavity (e.g., the bladder or the abdomen). For some types of skin cancer, chemotherapy can be applied as a cream or ointment directly to the skin.

Increasingly, chemotherapy can be given orally (by mouth), in the form of a tablet, capsule, or liquid. Patients commonly take oral chemotherapy at home. If you are responsible for administering your own chemotherapy, you must take it exactly as prescribed. If you are unable to do this, you need to notify your doctor immediately. Ask your doctor or nurse if you should follow any special instructions when handling chemotherapy at home.

Chemotherapy is given according to a schedule based on the type of cancer being treated and on the drugs being used. It may be given daily, weekly, every 2 to 3 weeks, or monthly. The schedule is often described as being in "cycles," with treatment for a defined period followed by a rest to allow the normal tissues of the body to recover from the effects of the chemotherapy. Chemotherapy may be given for a specific period of time (e.g., in six cycles) or indefinitely.

Diagnostic tests are ordered periodically during chemotherapy treatment. Some tests evaluate how the tumor is responding; for example, a CT, MRI, or bone scan may be ordered every 3 to 6 months to see if the tumor has gotten smaller, remained stable, or grown. Other tests evaluate how the normal tissues in your

Cancer and Cancer Treatment

body are responding, to ensure that the side effects of the treatment are not putting you at risk for further problems. For example, before each treatment, a **complete blood count (CBC)** may be ordered; this is a blood test to measure the number of white blood cells, red blood cells, and platelets. Its purpose is to check that your blood counts are not too low (see Question 35). Blood chemistries may be ordered to make sure your kidneys and liver are functioning normally (see Question 79).

Complete blood count (CBC)

A blood test to measure the number of white blood cells, red blood cells, and platelets.

7. What is targeted therapy?

Mary Ann's comment:

I am presently receiving targeted therapy in a clinical trial. Three years ago, my right upper lobe was removed as it contained a malignant stage 1, nonsmall cell tumor. I was fortunate in that there was no metastasis at that time, and, after careful consideration and several medical opinions, it was agreed that I did not need adjunct therapy of any kind. I was free of cancer—or so I thought.

For 2 years I diligently had my CT scans regularly. No sign of any cancer cells lurking. I began to relax and then in October 2008, almost 2 years to the day, my CT scan showed new growths in the right lung and what appeared to be a new cancer on the tail of my pancreas. Needless to say, I went into a complete panic.

Turned out that I was a rare case where the lung cells had traveled to the pancreas. This does not usually happen. It may seem very strange that I was so relieved to discover that I had lung cancer and not pancreatic cancer. Two days before Christmas 2008, I began a clinical trial with targeted therapy.

My big question—and fear—was how long would I be on this "trial" and if it didn't work, was I putting myself in jeop-

ardy? I was assured that if there was no improvement in 6 weeks, I would undergo a standard chemotherapy treatment.

I began taking 50 mg daily of this trial drug. My skin became very dry and I had a great deal of trouble with my intestines. The dosage was lowered to 40 mg and my skin improved except for a yeast infection under my breasts. This was handled with medication and flares occasionally. (I have to state that I've had this problem before I began the target medication as I am a large woman.) Eventually the dosage was moved to 30 mg, and I was given medication for my intestinal problems, which still persist. Around 5 months, I experienced some hair loss—ironically only the silver hair, and people thought I had colored my hair! I had a thick head of hair so most people don't notice the loss—I have to admit I do and I never realized how vain I was about my hair. I have to remind myself how lucky I am to be experiencing such minor side effects.

Within 6 weeks of taking this trial medication, the small growth on the pancreatic tail was no longer visible (and later referred to as "calcified"). At the 6-month mark, the small tumors in my right lung also seem to have responded favorably and are no longer visible.

It is my understanding that I will take this medication for the rest of my life. Isn't that a wonderful phrase, "the rest of my life"? Targeted therapy has given me hope that there is a long life ahead.

When treating cancers, doctors must now consider not only the origin of the cancer but also its biology. Recent laboratory research has helped us understand the complex biologic pathways in the cell that cause cancers to develop, grow, and spread. Targeted therapy works by blocking specific biologic pathways.

Targeted therapy works by blocking specific biologic pathways in the cell.

13

There are several classes of targeted therapies; each blocks a specific pathway. Here are examples from each class:

- Tyrosine kinase inhibitors
  - Tarceva (erlotinib)
  - Glivec (imatinib)
  - Herceptin (trastuzumab)
- Angiogenesis inhibitors
  - Avastin (bevacizumab)
- Proteosome inhibitors
  - Velcade (bortezomib)
- Targeted immunotherapy
  - Rituxan (rituximab)

Targeted therapy treatment affects only the cancer cells, having minimal effect on normal cells.

Targeted therapy treatment affects only the cancer cells, having minimal effect on normal cells. As an example of how targeted therapies work, angiogenesis inhibitors block the formation of new blood vessels. Cancer cells secrete proteins that promote the growth of new blood vessels, allowing the cells to multiply and spread. By blocking the formation of new tumor blood vessels, angiogenesis inhibitors prevent the cancer from growing, and the cancer cells are destroyed.

8. What types of biologic therapies are used to treat cancer?

Biologic therapy, also called biotherapy or immunotherapy, includes a wide variety of approaches that use the immune system to treat cancer. The immune system consists of special cells and chemicals with the ability to recognize and destroy foreign or abnormal cells, including cancer cells. Biologic therapy introduces human-made immune substances into the body. These substances can destroy the cancer cells, make the cells more vulnerable to destruction by the body's immune system, or strengthen the ability of the immune system to destroy the cancer cells.

Most biologic therapies are still experimental. They include:

- *Monoclonal antibodies:* These antibodies can recognize a specific abnormal protein on the surface of cancer cells, travel directly to these cells, and attack them. Examples of monoclonal antibodies used in cancer treatment are rituximab, trastuzumab, gemtuzumab, and alemtuzumab. These antibodies may be linked to chemotherapy or **radioactive isotopes** (unstable elements that emit radioactivity as they decay). The antibodies carry them to the site of cancer so the chemotherapy or radioactive isotopes can destroy the cancer cells. Because of their ability to differentiate between cancer cells and normal cells, monoclonal antibodies are a type of targeted therapy (see Question 7). An example of a monoclonal antibody linked to a radioactive isotope is ibritumomab tiuxetan.
- *Cytokines:* These chemicals can attack cancer cells or stimulate the immune system. Examples of cytokines used in cancer treatment are interferon, interleukin, and tumor necrosis factor.
- *Vaccines:* These are made from cancer cells that have been inactivated. Vaccines stimulate the immune system to make antibodies to destroy the cancer cells.

9. What types of hormonal therapies are used to treat cancer?

Hormones are chemicals produced by endocrine glands in the body. Cancer of the prostate and some cancers of the breast can be stimulated by specific hormones in the body. The hormones bind to receptors on the cancer cells' surface and stimulate the cells to multiply, causing the cancer to grow. Hormonal therapies stop the body from producing the hormones or block

Radioactive isotopes

Unstable elements that emit radioactivity as they decay (break down); used to take diagnostic images or to treat cancer.

Cancer and Cancer Treatment

their activity. The goal is to stop the cancer cells from dividing or to destroy them.

The male hormone testosterone, produced primarily by the testicles, stimulates prostate cancer to grow, and so hormonal therapy is one treatment for prostate cancer. Some medications, such as leuprolide and goserelin, stop the production of testosterone by the testicles. These medications, given by injection usually once a month or every 3 months, eliminate most of the testosterone in the body. Other medications given orally (e.g., flutamide, bicalutamide) may be given in addition to the injections to block the receptors on the prostate cancer cells, inactivating any remaining testosterone that is circulating.

Alternatively, the testicles may be surgically removed (*orchiectomy*) to prevent testosterone production, or the patient may be given female hormones (e.g., diethylstilbestrol) to counteract the effects of testosterone. Side effects of long-term hormonal therapy in men with prostate cancer may include hot flashes, breast swelling and tenderness, decreased sex drive, inability to have an erection, loss of bone mass (osteoporosis), fatigue, and metabolic changes leading to weight gain and an increased risk of diabetes and heart disease.

The female hormone estrogen, produced primarily by the ovaries, stimulates some types of breast cancer to grow, and hormonal therapy is therefore one treatment for breast cancer. The medication that has been used the longest is tamoxifen, an oral medication that blocks the receptors on the breast cancer cells. Other similar oral medications are raloxifene and toremifene. Fulvestrant, given by injection once a month, not only blocks the receptors; it also destroys them. Even after menopause, a woman's body produces a small amount of estrogen; a group of drugs called aromatase inhibitors (e.g., anastrozole, letrozole, exemestane) blocks the enzyme that stimulates this.

Alternatively, women may receive leuprolide injections to stop the production of estrogen by the ovaries, have their ovaries surgically removed, or be given the hormone megestrol. Side effects of hormonal therapy in women with breast cancer may include hot flashes, vaginal discharge or irritation, fatigue, visual changes, and an increased risk of developing endometrial cancer or ovarian cysts.

10. What are vascular access devices? Do I need one?

Receiving treatment for cancer often requires the nurse to frequently access your veins to draw blood, administer chemotherapy, or give intravenous fluids. The most common method is to insert a small metal or plastic needle under the skin into a vein in your hand or arm. Some people have veins that are difficult to find or that are very fragile, making visits to the doctor stressful because of worries that the nurse will not be able to get into the vein. In addition, some chemotherapy drugs are very irritating or must be given over many hours or days, with a risk that the drug can leak out of the vein and seep under your skin. To counteract these problems, special long-term vascular access devices have been developed to make it easier and safer for you to receive your treatment. These devices all have a special thin flexible catheter, or tube, that is placed under the skin and inserted into a large vein in your chest, leading to your heart. The catheter may be left in place for a number of months or years, until it is no longer needed.

In one type of device, the catheter is attached to an *implantable port*, a hollow round disk about the size of a

Special long-term vascular access devices have been developed to make it easier and safer for you to receive your treatment.

Cancer and Cancer Treatment

quarter and a half-inch high. The disk is placed under the skin, usually on the chest wall, under the collarbone. To access the device, the nurse inserts a special needle through the skin into the port. Between treatments, the nurse must flush the device once a month to prevent it from clotting, but no other care is required. If you are "needle phobic," ask your nurse about EMLA cream, which is a **topical anesthetic**. This medication can be applied to the skin directly over the port. The cream numbs the area, eliminating or reducing the pain of the needlestick. EMLA cream should be applied about 1 hour before your port is accessed.

Topical anesthetic

A medication applied to the surface of the body (for example, the skin or mucous membranes) to numb the area.

In another type of device, the catheter exits through the skin and is called an *external catheter*. Hickman catheters and PICC lines are examples of external catheters. The catheter may exit from the chest wall under the collarbone or on the arm. External catheters require frequent flushing and must be covered with a dressing. If you have an external catheter, your nurse will teach you how to take care of it. If you need a long-term catheter, your doctor will recommend the type that is best for you.

Long-term catheters can become infected and develop blood clots. Call your doctor immediately if you develop redness, swelling, discharge, or pain at the site of the port or where the catheter exits the skin, or if you develop swelling in the arm on the side of the catheter.

11. What are clinical trials?

Pete's comment:

I felt initially that one of the advantages of getting treatment at a cancer center was the potential of participating in a clinical research study. Every day you hear about new drugs that

*may have a positive effect on cancer, and I felt that partici-
pating in a trial was a good opportunity to take advantage of
the newest scientific research. When my treatment options
included a clinical trial, I didn't hesitate to participate.*

Mary Ann's comment:

*I am presently enrolled in a clinical trial—my diagnosis
fourth stage lung cancer. I was taken by surprise when my
lung cancer returned after 2 years. This time I went immediately to MSKCC [Memorial Sloan-Kettering Cancer
Center] for treatment.*

*Fortunately, I had a consultation there after my initial sur-
gery and in a study of my cancer cells, it appeared that I
carried a mutated gene on my cancer cells. I was asked if I
would consider being part of a clinical trial team that was
treating this type of cancer.*

*Not without some trepidation—I feared being given a
placebo, but with my family urging me to take part in this—I
decided that it was worth a try. I was also assured that there
were no "blind" studies and that no one in the study would be
given a placebo. I was also assured that if there was no sign of
improvement in 6 weeks, I would be taken out of the trial
and put on a more conventional form of chemotherapy.*

*As part of the clinical trial, I am carefully monitored. For
the first few months, I was tested every 2 weeks—blood,
urine, scans, EKG, etc. Progress was swift for me and
within 6 weeks, a tiny growth on the tail of my pancreas
(which was an unusual form of the lung cancer metastasis)
had calcified and was no longer an issue. I am just past
6 months in the trial, and the growths in my lungs seem to
have also shrunk to nothing.*

*When I began this trial, I thought back to my days in
kindergarten—I was one of the children given the Salk
vaccine for polio in that "clinical trial." Months later, we*

were notified that I had indeed received the live vaccine. I felt heroic as a child—and I feel heroic now. Regardless of how this turns out in the long run, I feel as though it gives my life purpose and if it doesn't work for me, it may be the building block for someone else in the future.

In one irony of this, the medication I am on has helped my arthritis and literally cured my diabetes. My blood sugar has been normal—with no medication—since the trial began. Who knows what other benefits may come from this trial?

Clinical trials are research studies designed to test new treatments on humans. Any kind of treatment may be studied—methods of administering radiation therapy, drugs (including chemotherapy), biologic agents, nutritional therapies, medical devices, or even behavioral therapies. Either a single new treatment or standard treatments combined in new ways may be studied.

New treatments are usually first developed in a laboratory and then tested on animals. If they seem to provide some benefit, they are tested in phases on humans to determine their safety and effectiveness.

- *Phase I* clinical trials are undertaken first, to determine the appropriate dose and schedule for the treatment, as well as its side effects.
- *Phase II* clinical trials test the treatment on patients with a particular type of cancer to determine effectiveness.
- *Phase III* clinical trials are conducted on patients with a particular type of cancer to compare the effectiveness of the new treatment with that of the standard treatment. Half the patients in the study get the new treatment and half get the standard treatment.

Patients enrolled in a Phase III clinical trial are randomly assigned to be in one of these groups. You cannot select the treatment you want.

Participating in a clinical trial is not being a "guinea pig." The studies are designed thoughtfully and are based on information previously learned about the new treatment. To protect the safety of patients, the U.S. Food and Drug Administration (FDA) strictly regulates and monitors how clinical trials are conducted. The study must undergo internal review at the hospital the doctor is affiliated with, and it must be approved and monitored by an Institutional Review Board (IRB). In addition, for each study, very specific **eligibility criteria** describe who can be treated in the study; these criteria consist of a list of conditions that must be met for someone to enroll in a clinical trial. Finally, a clinical trial requires a **consent form**, a written document signed by patients to indicate that they have been informed about a treatment, as well as the associated risks and benefits, and that they agree to receive the treatment. The form describes the purpose of the study, the treatment the participants will receive, the possible side effects, the risks and benefits, and the financial costs. Before receiving any treatment, you must sign this consent form, indicating that you understand the study and you agree to participate in it.

Participating in a clinical trial gives you the opportunity to receive new treatments before they are available to other people. You receive care by a leading doctor affiliated with a major cancer center, and you are closely monitored throughout your treatment. You also contribute to progress in medical science. Just remember that the treatment given in a clinical trial is not yet proven to be more effective than the standard treatment

To protect patients, the U.S. Food and Drug Administration strictly regulates and monitors clinical trials.

Eligibility criteria

A list of conditions that must be met for someone to enroll in a clinical trial.

Consent form

A written document signed by patients to indicate that they have been informed about a treatment, as well as the associated risks and benefits, and that they agree to receive the treatment; also referred to as *informed consent*.

you might otherwise receive, and you could even have unexpected side effects. Furthermore, you may have to spend more time receiving treatment, having the required diagnostic tests, and seeing the doctor. In addition, the financial cost to you may be greater. Your health insurance might not cover some aspects of the care, and you might have to pay for transportation or housing if the treatment is not close to home.

Although most cancer clinical trials are designed to test new treatments for cancer, an increasing number of trials are designed to test new methods of managing the symptoms experienced by people with cancer. If you are interested in finding out more about clinical trials, an excellent source of information is *Taking Part in Clinical Trials: What Cancer Patients Need to Know*, a booklet available from the Cancer Information Service of the National Cancer Institute. To find out how to find a clinical trial that might be appropriate for you, see Question 17.

12. What are complementary and alternative treatments?

Complementary and alternative medicine (CAM) includes a wide variety of approaches to improving health and treating disease that the traditional medical community does not recognize as standard or conventional. When used in addition to conventional methods of treatment, they are referred to as *complementary*; when used instead of conventional methods of treatment, they are referred to as *alternative*.

Complementary and alternative therapies may be categorized in many different ways. The National Center for Complementary and Alternative Medicine (NCCAM) divides them into five domains:

1. *Whole medical systems of theory and practice:* These are practices used by different cultures in various parts of the world to stimulate or support the body's ability to heal itself or restore the yin-yang balance and flow of qi. Examples include *homeopathic medicine, naturopathic medicine,* traditional Chinese medicine (e.g., **acupuncture**), and Ayurveda.

2. *Mind–body medicine:* These techniques help the mind enhance body functions and reduce symptoms. Examples include meditation, guided imagery, hypnosis, prayer, and creative therapies.

3. *Biologically based practices:* These use substances found in nature such as herbs, foods, vitamins, and other biologic products (e.g., shark cartilage).

4. *Manipulative and body-based practices:* These techniques involve the manipulation or movement of the body, such as those used by chiropractors and massage therapists.

5. *Energy medicine:* These techniques manipulate energy fields within or outside the body. Examples include therapeutic touch, the use of magnets, or *Reiki* (a technique of placing hands lightly on the body or just above it to heal the spirit and thus the body).

Acupuncture
A technique of inserting thin needles into the body at specific locations with the goal of restoring the normal flow of energy in the body; often used to treat pain or other symptoms.

The practice of complementary and alternative therapies is rapidly increasing, partly due to our increasing understanding of them. The body of scientific knowledge about specific complementary and alternative therapies, how they work, and what effects they have on the body is constantly growing. To disseminate authoritative information about complementary and alternative therapies and to scientifically study their safety and effectiveness, the U.S. government founded the National

Cancer and Cancer Treatment

Center for Complementary and Alternative Medicine as part of the National Institutes of Health.

However, the increased use of such therapies also reflects the desperation of many people with cancer, resulting in a willingness to try anything and everything they feel might help them. Complementary and alternative therapies are not regulated in the same way as traditional medications and medical devices. Many treatments and products offer no evidence of effectiveness, and, in fact, some may even be harmful to you. If you are considering unconventional therapies, get as much accurate information as you can about them. Discuss your thoughts with your doctor, and inform him or her of your intentions. Many of these therapies can be used safely with the traditional treatments you are receiving. Others, however, can interfere with your treatment, cause serious side effects when combined with your treatment, or may even be harmful to you. See Question 18 to learn how to obtain additional information about complementary and alternative therapies.

If you are considering unconventional therapies, get as much accurate information as you can about them, and speak with your doctor before you begin.

13. Why do cancer treatments cause side effects? Is my treatment more likely to work if I get more severe side effects?

Despite the most careful precautions for treating a cancer safely, most treatments cause side effects. For many types of cancer, surgery to remove the tumor is an important part of the treatment. However, depending on the type of cancer and the extent of surgery performed, there may be changes in how your body looks or functions. Chemotherapy and radiation therapy work primarily by attacking the cancer cell's ability to divide. Because normal cells also need to divide for the body to function normally, they may also be damaged by treatment, causing side effects. Radiation therapy and some types of chemotherapy may also injure organs in the body.

Some side effects occur during or shortly after treatment and resolve completely after treatment is completed. *Acute* or *early side effects* generally resolve within weeks or a few months after treatment is completed Examples are drops in blood counts, nausea, vomiting, diarrhea, and mouth sores. *Long-term side effects* may persist for months or years after treatment. Examples are nerve damage or fatigue. *Late side effects* may not show up for months or years after treatment is completed. Examples are infertility, heart or lung problems, or cataracts. Although these are rarer than early or long-term effects, these are permanent and can cause significant problems.

Planning treatment for any one person always involves balancing the risks of treatment with the potential benefits. Your doctor will discuss these with you before you begin treatment so that you understand the goals of treatment and the potential side effects you may experience.

A common myth is that the severity of side effects indicates the effectiveness of treatment. Some people might even avoid taking medication to relieve their side effects, thinking that their treatment will work better. This is not true. Some people who have successful treatment with a long-term cure have minimal side effects. Unfortunately, others have very severe side effects during treatment, even requiring hospitalization, and yet their cancer does not respond to treatment and continues to grow and spread.

The severity of side effects is usually linked to the type of treatment you are receiving. Some treatments are known to cause significant side effects; others are very

Cancer and Cancer Treatment

Planning treatment always involves balancing the risks with the potential benefits.

The severity of side effects is usually linked to the type of treatment you are receiving.

well tolerated. Your general state of health, your level of activity, and how well you are eating and drinking can also affect how you tolerate treatment. Taking medication to manage side effects does not interfere with the treatment. In fact, it helps you feel better so that you can eat and drink well and maintain your usual activities as much as possible.

Lisa's comment:

Even though I uttered the word myth *countless times to my own patients, when I experienced minimal side effects from chemotherapy and radiation therapy (at first) I found myself thinking: "I wonder if this is working!" Intellectually, I knew it was, but emotionally. . . . Funny.*

14. How does my doctor evaluate whether my treatment is working? What if my treatment doesn't work?

During regular visits throughout your treatment, your doctor evaluates how you are doing. These visits are necessary to see how you are tolerating the treatment, if you are having side effects, and, if so, how severe they are. The doctor may order medication to relieve the side effects and may even make adjustments in your treatment dose or schedule. Another reason for these visits is to see how your cancer is responding to the treatment. If you have had the cancer removed by surgery or destroyed by chemotherapy or radiation therapy, the doctor wants to be sure that the cancer has not recurred (reappeared). If the cancer could not be removed or destroyed, the doctor wants to be sure it is not progressing (growing) or metastasizing (spreading to other areas). The doctor reviews any symptoms you are having and performs a physical examination. Blood tests are done, and at periodic intervals radiologic studies, such as CT, MRI, or PET, are performed to see images of the body. The specific types of studies depend on the type of cancer you have.

If you are tolerating treatment well and there is no sign that the disease has recurred, progressed, or metastasized, your doctor will continue the treatment. Depending on your situation, the treatment may be planned for a defined period of time (e.g., 6 months) or given indefinitely. However, if you develop a recurrence or if the tumor progresses or metastasizes while you are on treatment, the cancer cells may have become resistant to the treatment you are getting. If so, your doctor will recommend discontinuing your current treatment and discuss other options with you. If your energy level is good, if your weight is fairly stable, and if you are able to be up and around most of the day, you are more likely to have a good response to active treatment, so your doctor will probably recommend a new type of treatment.

If you have been hoping for a cure, hearing that your disease has recurred or spread is distressing. You may find yourself experiencing again many of the feelings you had when you were first diagnosed: anger, sadness, worry, or even difficulty accepting the reality of what the doctor is telling you. You may feel frightened that you will develop new physical symptoms. You may feel concerned about family and friends. You may be worried about the financial implications for your family. You may feel spiritually distressed.

If you have been hoping for a cure, hearing that your disease has recurred or spread is distressing. There are ways to cope.

There are ways to cope. Questions 88–90 have suggestions on how to cope with these emotions and concerns.

Getting accurate information from your doctor is particularly important as you consider what comes next.

Some people find it helpful to have their doctor fully explain the details of their illness and prognosis. Others prefer not to hear the details and just focus on the plan. Decide what you want to know and communicate this to your family and doctor (see Question 16).

In making decisions about treatment if your cancer recurs or spreads, talk with your doctor about the goal of the treatment being recommended. Consider whether this matches your own goals. Talk with your family and doctor about what is most important to you at this time in your life. A resource that may be helpful during this time is *When Cancer Returns*, published by the National Cancer Institute.

15. What happens after my cancer treatment is completed? How do I adjust to being a survivor?

Completing treatment for cancer and becoming a survivor bring new challenges.

Completing treatment for cancer and becoming a survivor bring new challenges. When your treatment is completed, your doctor will schedule regular follow-up visits to be sure you are recovering from treatment, to make sure you have not developed any long-term side effects from treatment, and to evaluate the status of your tumor. Your doctor will ask about symptoms, perform a physical examination, draw blood for laboratory analysis, and order radiologic studies, such as CT, MRI, or PET. The specific blood tests and radiologic studies depend on the type of cancer you have. These studies help the doctor determine whether the tumor has grown back (recurrence) or cells have begun to grow in other parts of the body (metastasis). If all the tests are negative, if you have no signs or symptoms of cancer, and if there is "no evidence of disease," the doctor may say you are in **remission**. When these circumstances continue over a number of years, the doctor may say you are *cured*.

Remission

A disappearance of all signs and symptoms of cancer.

Initially, your doctor may want to see you every 2 to 3 months. Over time, the visits will be farther apart, going to every 6 months and then to once a year. If you have received combined treatments, clarify with your doctors—your surgeon, medical oncologist (who prescribes chemotherapy), and radiation oncologist (who prescribes radiation therapy)—when you should see each of them.

For many people, the days immediately before their doctor's appointments and the days waiting for the results of diagnostic tests are times of anxiety and worry. Completing treatment for cancer brings other challenges as well. Among these may be adjusting to changes in your body, recovering strength after treatment, resuming your usual activities, returning to work, and explaining your illness to friends and colleagues. In addition, despite the fact that your treatment is over, you may find it difficult at times to balance the hopefulness that the disease will not come back with the knowledge that the future is always uncertain. Each of these challenges presents a new hurdle to overcome. Give yourself time as you transition into feeling "normal" again. Draw on your usual methods of coping, as well as those you learned after your diagnosis and during your treatment (see Question 92).

Three resources may be helpful to you as you adjust to your life as a cancer survivor:

1. *Facing Forward Series: Life After Cancer Treatment*, published by the National Cancer Institute, covers post-treatment issues such as follow-up medical care, physical and emotional changes, changes in social relationships, and workplace issues.
2. The Cancer Survivors Network of the American Cancer Society (www.acscsn.org) offers recorded

discussions on issues and provides an opportunity to interact with other survivors.

3. The National Coalition for Cancer Survivorship (www.canceradvocacy.org), an advocacy organization for cancer survivors, has valuable information, including a Cancer Survival Toolbox.

Despite the fears and uncertainties, some people find that being diagnosed with cancer gives them the opportunity to think about their lives in new ways. Relationships often become stronger and enriched by the experience. Sometimes people choose to shift the priorities in their life, ensuring that they are spending their time doing what is most important to them.

Mary Ann's comment:

After my cancer treatment was completed 3 years ago, my oncologist followed up with CT scans on a scheduled basis—first year, every 3 months; second year, every 6 months. There were also follow-up blood and urine tests. Fortunately for me, the CT scan picked up a recurrence of my cancer at the 2-year marker. Tiny tumors appeared in the lining of my right lung and on the tail of my pancreas. It was a very scary time for me and my family. However, because of the good follow-up care, these tumors were caught at a very early stage and I was fortunate enough to be eligible for a clinical trial at Memorial Sloan-Kettering Cancer Center. I am in my 8th month of this trial and today I can say that it appears that my tumors have shrunk and calcified. Am I out of the woods permanently? Probably not but with good follow-up care, I expect to live for a long time!

PART TWO

Getting Information and Making Decisions

How can I be sure to get the information
I want from my doctor?

How can I find clinical trials that may
be appropriate for me?

I feel so overwhelmed by all the information
I'm getting. How do I make decisions
about my treatment?

More . . .

16. How can I be sure to get the information I want from my doctor?

Pete's comment:

Before meeting with my oncologist, I write my questions on an index card. My wife is always with me to ask additional questions and take notes if necessary. By using this approach, I feel much more relaxed and in control. I also find that my oncologist's nurse practitioner is extremely helpful and provides follow-up answers to a number of questions.

Mary Ann's comment:

It is very important to establish a good rapport with your doctor and the nurses who care for us. We have to realize that these medical professionals want what is best for us. However, we do not always hear what we are being told, and it is important to bring along someone who will remain objective and keep track of the information given to you by the medical staff and prompt you to ask the questions that you always think of after you leave the doctor's office. Don't be afraid to ask any question regarding your care. It's far better for the staff to know what is on your mind so that they can put you at ease with whatever decisions you make.

It's important to feel comfortable with your doctor, to trust his or her medical judgment, and to feel you can communicate. Doctors will generally try to tell you everything you *need* to know about your disease and treatment, but they may not tell you everything you *want* to know. So, first, you must decide what you want to know.

Everyone approaches a diagnosis of cancer differently. Some people want to know every detail about their disease, treatment, and prognosis and to be involved in every decision. Others prefer to know only the basics and to have their family or doctor make the decisions for them. Of course, many people fall between these extremes. In addition, at various points in time, you may want to know different things. When you are first diagnosed, your concerns will be different from those you may have during treatment or when you are no longer receiving treatment.

Each time you visit your doctor, decide beforehand what questions you have. Talk with members of your family or anyone else you can speak openly with to focus your thoughts and concerns. Write your questions down on a piece of paper. There are no stupid questions, so include everything that concerns you. When you see your doctor, state at the beginning of the visit that, before you leave that day, you would like to ask questions. That helps your doctor plan extra time to speak with you. Here are some questions you may want to ask when you first meet with your oncologist:

Before each visit with your doctor, write your questions down on a piece of paper.

- Is the cancer localized, or has it spread to other sites?
- What other diagnostic tests do I need?
- Can this cancer be surgically removed?
- What choices do I have to treat the cancer?
- What treatment do you recommend and why?
- What is the goal of this treatment?
- What are the risks of this treatment?
- How will you know if the treatment is working?
- What are the alternatives to this treatment?
- How will I feel during and after treatment?
- What side effects will I have from treatment?
- What are the possible long-term effects of treatment?
- What do I need to do to care for myself during treatment?

Getting Information and Making Decisions

33

- Will I be able to work and continue my usual activities during treatment?
- For what reasons should I call your office?

When answering your questions, your doctor may present a lot of information and use terms that are unfamiliar or confusing. As you listen, you may feel anxious or afraid and find it difficult to understand everything that is being said. If you don't understand something, ask the doctor to explain it.

If you don't understand something, ask the doctor to explain it.

You may find it helpful to bring a family member or friend with you to your doctor visits. They can be a second set of ears, can take notes while the doctor is speaking, and can review the answers with you when you get home. If something is still unclear when you get home, call the office the next day. The nurse who works with your doctor may also be able to answer many of your questions. You are entitled to have your questions answered; be persistent.

Some patients find they are more comfortable not getting detailed answers to questions, but family members may have many questions. Identify one person to be the family spokesperson, coming to office visits and contacting your doctor as needed to ask questions. The family spokesperson can use the same suggestions just described to clarify what everyone wants to know and to be sure to get everyone's questions answered.

17. How can I find clinical trials that may be appropriate for me?

Clinical trials

Research studies to test the effectiveness of new treatments on humans.

Clinical trials are research studies designed to test the effectiveness of new treatments on humans (see Question 11). If you are interested in participating in a clinical trial, hold off starting treatment until you have investigated the options. Ask your doctor for recommendations and whether it is safe for you to delay your treatment. Your doctor may also be able to help you find clinical trials available for you and determine whether you are eligible for them.

The following resources provide listings of clinical trials for particular cancers and cancer symptoms:

- *National Cancer Institute:* www.cancer.gov/clinicaltrials or 800-4-CANCER
- *National Institutes of Health:* www.clinicaltrials.gov
- *Coalition of Cancer Cooperative Groups:* www.cancertrialshelp.org or 877-520-4457
- *Centerwatch:* www.centerwatch.com
- *National Comprehensive Cancer Network (NCCN):* www.nccn.org (Select "Find a Member Institution" to find a cancer center in your geographic region. Contact them to see if any clinical trials are available for you.)

18. How can I find out about complementary or alternative therapies?

Complementary and alternative medicine (CAM) refers to a wide variety of approaches to improving health and treating disease that the traditional medical community does not recognize as standard or conventional. When used in addition to conventional methods of treatment, they are referred to as *complementary*; when used instead of conventional methods of treatment, they are referred to as *alternative* (see Question 12).

There are several reliable sources of information about complementary and alternative therapies. Because of the rapidly changing state of knowledge about this area of medicine, the Internet provides the most up-to-date information. The following websites provide general information on these therapies:

- *Cancer Information Service of the National Cancer Institute:* www.cancer.gov/cancerinfo/treatment/cam
- *National Center for Complementary and Alternative Medicine of the National Institutes of Health:* www.nccam.nih.gov/health
- *Memorial Sloan–Kettering Cancer Center:* www.mskcc.org/aboutherbs
- *MD Anderson Cancer Center:* www.mdanderson.org/topics/complementary
- *The Richard and Hinda Rosenthal Center for Complementary and Alternative Medicine:* www.rosenthal.hs.columbia.edu
- *American Academy of Medical Acupuncture:* www.medicalacupuncture.org

The following organizations provide information specifically on dietary supplements, including vitamins, minerals, and **botanicals** (plants or plant parts valued for their medicinal properties; includes herbal products; commonly prepared as a tea, an extract, or a tincture):

- *Office of Dietary Supplements of the National Institutes of Health:* www.dietary-supplements.info.nih.gov
- *Center for Food Safety and Applied Nutrition of the U.S. Food and Drug Administration:* www.cfsan.fda.gov
- *American Botanical Council:* www.herbalgram.org

Finally, for scientific bibliographic citations related to particular therapies, see the

- *National Library of Medicine:* www.nlm.nih.gov/nccam/camonpubmed.html

Botanicals

Plants or plant parts valued for their medicinal properties; includes herbal products; commonly prepared as a tea, an extract, or a tincture.

19. How do I decide whether to use one of the complementary or alternative therapies that my family or friends is recommending?

Before beginning treatment with any complementary or alternative therapy, obtain as much information as you can about it. Question 18 provides suggestions on how to do that. Here are some specific questions to consider:

- Do the promises sound too good to be true, such as promises that are inconsistent with the information you are receiving from your doctor or from other sources of information?
- What evidence supports the claims of effectiveness? Were scientific, rigorously controlled clinical trials conducted? Or is the evidence only *anecdotal*, that is, based on the author's personal experience or claims of satisfied customers?
- What are the risks of using this treatment? What is the evidence regarding safety? How are data collected to evaluate safety?
- If someone is providing the therapy, what are the person's qualifications, certifications, or licenses? Some practitioners are now licensed by state medical boards or accredited by professional organizations.
- Is the source of information about the therapy also the seller? If so, the seller may have a vested interest in convincing you to purchase the product.

Two Internet sites provide tips to help with decisions about using a complementary or alternative therapy:

- *National Center for Complementary and Alternative Medicine of the National Institutes of Health:* www. nccam.nih.gov/health/decisions/index.htm

Getting Information and Making Decisions

- Center for Food Safety and Applied Nutrition of the U.S. Food and Drug Administration: www.cfsan.fda.gov/~dms/ds-savvy.html

Before making a final decision about the use of any complementary or alternative therapy, discuss your thoughts and intentions with your doctor.

Before making a final decision about the use of any complementary or alternative therapy, discuss your thoughts and intentions with your doctor. Many of these therapies can be used safely with the traditional treatments you are receiving. However, some can interfere with your treatment, cause serious side effects when combined with your treatment, or may actually be harmful.

20. How can I evaluate information on the Internet to be sure it is complete, accurate, and up-to-date?

Pete's comment:

The sheer amount of information on the Internet can be intimidating and confusing. By concentrating on several credible and reputable sites, I get good background data, which increase my knowledge without overwhelming me. I also find that cancer center websites are a good source of information. If I have questions, I refer to my oncology team for clarification.

Because the information posted on the Internet is not controlled or regulated, a great deal of it may not be accurate.

The Internet has created the opportunity for you to get instant access to an enormous amount of information without ever leaving your home. However, because the information posted on the Internet is not controlled or regulated, a great deal of it may not be accurate.

When viewing a site, a number of things can help you determine whether it is reliable and likely to have complete, accurate, and up-to-date information:

- *Ownership or sponsorship of the site:* The owner or sponsor of the site pays for it to be maintained. The owner or sponsor may be a government agency, a nonprofit organization, a medical center or hospital, a pharmaceutical company, or an individual. The sponsor can influence what content is presented. Consider whether the sponsor may benefit by presenting a biased point of view.
- *Purpose of the site:* Click on "About this site." The site's purpose should be clearly stated and will help determine whether it has a particular point of view.
- *Editorial board:* Many sites have an editorial board that reviews all the information posted. Review the list of people on the editorial board, and check their credentials and affiliations to be sure they are medically qualified to make these decisions.
- *Source of information:* The authors of the information should be identified. Review their credentials and affiliations to be sure they are truly experts in the field. If the information is obtained from other sources, these also should be acknowledged.
- *Evidence:* References to scientific research findings and published articles that back up the information should be included.
- *The date information was updated:* The site should include a statement indicating the date the information was last reviewed and updated. Medical information must be current to be useful.
- *Privacy:* The site may ask for information about you. If so, it should clearly state how the information will be used and how your privacy will be protected.

Before acting on any information you have obtained from the Internet, discuss what you have found and what you are considering with your doctor.

21. I feel so overwhelmed by all the information I'm getting. How do I make decisions about my treatment?

Pete's comment:

After receiving my lung cancer diagnosis, my wife and I were overwhelmed. We decided to take it one step at a time and move slowly. The first thing we felt was necessary was to get a second opinion at another institution. Our primary concern was being comfortable with the oncologist and his medical team. We also were very aware of the proximity of the potential treatment center and if the treatment was covered by my medical insurance.

After being diagnosed with cancer, one of the most stressful periods of time is when you have to make decisions about your treatment. A number of things can help you sort out the available options and select the best one for you.

First, be sure you have all the relevant information. Are you clear about your clinical situation and the choices being presented to you? If not, refer to Question 16 for suggestions on how to obtain the information you need from your doctors.

Second, be sure you have seen all the treating specialists to hear their recommendations directly. **Internists** (physicians who specialize in the diagnosis and medical treatment of adults) or surgeons can provide you with direction, but they will not be able to give you detailed information about chemotherapy or radiation therapy. If these treatments are being recommended, schedule appointments with a medical oncologist (who prescribes chemotherapy) and a radiation oncologist (who prescribes radiation therapy). Clarify with each doctor

Internists

Physicians who specialize in the diagnosis and medical treatment of adults.

the goals of treatment. Also ask about the potential side effects or risks of treatment. See Question 16 for a list of additional questions you may want to ask. This approach will help you weigh the choices for yourself.

Once you are clear on the options posed by your doctors, consider whether it would be worthwhile to obtain a second opinion, perhaps with a specialist at an academic center or comprehensive cancer center. Doctors who specialize in treating particular types of cancer have more experience with this disease and may have a different perspective about treatment. In addition, they may be able to offer you treatment on a clinical trial.

Have a family member or friend accompany you to all these appointments. They can provide a second set of ears to hear the information presented and take notes for you while the doctors are speaking. When you get home, you will also have someone to review all the information with you to be sure you understand it correctly.

In making your final treatment decision, consider several other factors. Financial issues are important.

- What are the costs of the various treatment options, including treatment on a clinical trial?
- Does your health insurance cover treatment by any doctor or only by doctors affiliated with your health insurance plan?
- Will treatment on a clinical trial be covered?
- What percentage of the costs will be reimbursed to you and what will be the out-of-pocket expenses?

Getting Information and Making Decisions

Logistical issues are also important.

- Where would you have to go for treatment?
- Will it be easy to get back and forth, or will you have to travel long distances or even relocate to a different city for a period of time?

Finally, consider your emotional reactions to the doctors you have met.

- Did you feel you could trust the doctor and his or her medical team?
- Did you feel you were given adequate time to have all your questions answered?
- Did you feel treated respectfully and courteously by the staff in the office?

It is important to feel comfortable with the doctor you choose, because the two of you will be partners in the journey that lies ahead.

In the end, it comes down to you. Consider everything about your current life situation: how old you are; your general state of health; your responsibilities to your family and work; the emotional, physical, and financial costs of treatment; and all that you may possibly gain from treatment. The most difficult part of this process is that there is no right decision other than the one that feels right to you.

There is no right decision other than the one that feels right to you.

22. I want to have the best quality of life possible. Should I refuse to take any treatment so I won't have side effects?

One of the most difficult aspects of being diagnosed with cancer is living with uncertainty about the future. Coupled with that is the fear of side effects from treatment. These feelings can lead to questioning whether it is worthwhile to get treatment. But your decisions about treatment should be based on knowledge, not on fear. Speak with your doctor to get the information you need.

The side effects and the likelihood of long-term control or cure are based on the type of cancer you have, on the stage of disease, and on the treatment you receive. Everyone responds differently to treatment; no one can predict precisely what will happen to you. However, your doctor can explain what he or she hopes to achieve and what you will most likely experience during and after treatment. Consider this information when making your decision.

When a cancer is curable, making the decision is relatively easy because the goal is easy to understand. Many treatments are easily tolerated, with minimal disruption in your usual routines, and many side effects from the treatment resolve without any long-term consequences.

Even for those who cannot be cured, obtaining treatment offers a number of benefits. Many types of cancer can be controlled with treatment for a long period of time, even for a number of years. Equally important, treatment can improve the quality of your life. It can lessen or prevent symptoms of the disease, and it can prevent or delay complications from the growth of the cancer.

For specific questions to ask your doctor to ensure you get the information you need to make the decision about undergoing treatment for your cancer, see Question 16.

23. What is palliative care and how can I get referred to a palliative care program?

Palliative care addresses the medical, physical, emotional, social, and spiritual needs of patients to help them achieve the best possible quality of life. Historically,

Your decisions about treatment should be based on knowledge, not on fear.

Getting Information and Making Decisions

Palliative care

A philosophy of care that helps patients achieve the best possible quality of life.

43

palliative care was associated with hospice care and was reserved for patients at the end of life who were no longer receiving active treatment for their disease. However, in recent years the focus of palliative care has expanded to include all patients who could benefit from this approach, even those receiving active treatment and with a good prognosis. Many hospitals have established palliative care programs for their patients.

Although oncologists have a great deal of experience in managing pain and other symptoms, for some patients the usual interventions are not effective. In these cases, a referral to a palliative care specialist may be helpful. *Palliative care specialists* are physicians who are specially trained in techniques to manage pain and other symptoms.

If you feel your pain or other symptoms are not adequately controlled, ask your doctor about seeing a palliative care specialist. An Internet site that can provide additional information about palliative care and help you find a nearby provider is Get Palliative Care (www.getpalliativecare.org/home).

24. What are advance directives? How can I be sure my wishes are known?

Advance directives

Legal documents in which you indicate who you want to make medical decisions for you and/or what type of medical care you want to receive if you become unable to make decisions or speak for yourself in the future.

Advance directives are legal documents in which you indicate who you want to make medical decisions for you and/or what type of medical care you want to receive if you become unable to make decisions or speak for yourself in the future. Although the specific laws and terminology for advance directives vary from state to state, there are two basic types:

• A living will
• A health care proxy

A **living will** is a document in which you state specific instructions regarding your health care, outlining which medical interventions you want to have performed and which you want to have withheld, given a variety of circumstances. For example, if you were to lose the ability to eat and drink, would you want to receive artificial nutrition through a feeding tube or by means of intravenous fluids? If your heart were to stop beating, would you want to have your chest compressed or have your heart shocked? If you were to stop breathing, would you want a tube placed down your throat and connected to a respirator, which would breathe for you?

When making these decisions, specify the circumstances in which you want your wishes followed. If the medical problem is treatable and reversible, you may want all medical measures taken to resuscitate and support you. If the medical problem results from progressive cancer that can no longer be controlled, you may not want any aggressive measures taken to resuscitate you or to prolong your life. Deciding not to accept aggressive care to prolong your life is not the same as withholding other medical care. You can still receive pain medication, antibiotics, food and fluid, and other supportive measures. However, the goal of treatment shifts from cure to comfort care.

Making these decisions is very difficult, and you need to think about what you want for yourself. A living will provides you the opportunity to state your decisions so that people can act on them.

One significant limitation to a living will is that you can't foresee all possible health-related circumstances. Decisions might have to be made that you have not specified in writing. These problems can be avoided by

Living will

A document in which you can state specific instructions regarding your health care, outlining which medical interventions you want to have performed and which you want to have withheld, given a variety of circumstances.

Getting Information and Making Decisions

completing another legal document called a *health care proxy*, or *durable power of attorney for health care*. This document allows you to designate a **health care agent**, who is a person designated to make health care decisions for you if you are not able to. The designated person acts as your agent, deciding which medical interventions should be performed and which should be withheld. Although the terminology varies from state to state, all states recognize a health care proxy.

Health care agent

A person designated to make health care decisions for you if you are not able to.

When selecting a health care agent, be sure to choose among people you trust, those who will make decisions based on what you want for yourself, not on what they want for you or on what they would want for themselves if they were in your position. You can choose your health care agent among family members or friends. Talk with candidates about what you want for yourself in a variety of circumstances. Talk about the issues just described with regard to resuscitation and life-prolonging measures like artificial nutrition and intravenous fluid. Be as specific as you can be. Then confirm with the person you choose that he or she will honor your wishes and be willing to speak for you. You can change your health care agent, as well as your decisions about what you want done, at any time.

Let your family and friends know whom you have selected as your agent so that, if the need arises, everyone can support the person in making the necessary decisions. If you have completed a living will, share this with the family as well. Inform all of your doctors and everyone else on your medical team of your wishes and provide them with copies of any advance directive documents you have signed.

Having a discussion about what you would want if you were unable to make decisions for yourself is difficult for most people. Sometimes the patient wants to bring up the subject but is afraid the family will be distressed by the conversation. Sometimes the family wants to bring it up but is afraid of alarming the patient. It is always better to talk about these things when you are feeling well and when no imminent crisis is looming. With this type of preparation, you can calmly think about what you want and clearly talk about it with others.

You can initiate the discussion in several ways. You could say something like, "I want to be sure that, if I were to become sicker, you would know what I want done." A family member could initiate the discussion by saying something like, "If you were to become sicker and couldn't tell me what kind of care you wanted, I wouldn't know what to do. Can we talk about this?" Some people find that their family does not agree with the decisions they have made, making a difficult discussion even harder. This makes it all the more important to have an advance directive to ensure your wishes will be honored.

You can obtain state-specific advance directive documents from your lawyer, your doctor, your local hospital, or Caring Connections (http://www.caringinfo.org/stateaddownload).

PART THREE

Comfort, Activity, and Sleep

Will I have pain? What are the options available to treat my pain?

I feel tired much of the time. What can I do to increase my energy?

Can I exercise?

More . . .

COPING WITH PAIN

25. Will I have pain? What are the options available to treat my pain?

Pete's comment:

When I was first diagnosed, I had peripheral pain, which would flare up in my back throughout the day. I was put on Tylenol 3 (acetaminophen with codeine) to help manage it. This worked well and after several sessions of chemotherapy, the pain subsided and I was able to cut back on the medication. Eventually, the pain disappeared completely.

Pain has long been considered an unavoidable consequence of having cancer. However, with new pain medications and a better understanding of how to use them effectively, cancer pain can be well controlled in almost all people.

Not everyone with cancer develops pain. If a tumor grows or spreads, it may press on or invade surrounding organs or nerves. Depending on the location of the tumor, this pressure may cause pain. In addition, procedures used to diagnose or treat cancer may cause pain, such as having a biopsy to take a sample of tissue for diagnosing the type of cancer or having surgery to remove all or part of a tumor.

Pain may be experienced in many different ways, for example, discomfort, aching, a gnawing feeling, a sharp stabbing sensation, or cramping. Pain may be mild or severe, and it may be intermittent or continuous.

Many people are concerned about taking pain medication. Some feel that withstanding the pain is a sign of strength. Some people feel it is a part of having cancer that they have to accept. Some people are afraid of "masking" a problem—if they treat the pain, they think their doctor will not be able to follow their response to treatment. There is no benefit at all to having pain. Regardless of how mild it is, chronic pain can be very disabling. It affects your energy level, your appetite, your ability to sleep, your desire to be with friends and family, and your mood. Tell your doctor or nurse about any discomfort you have, no matter how mild. Try to describe it accurately so that they can decide on the best treatment for you and monitor the effectiveness of the treatment. When describing your discomfort, include the following information:

- Where you feel the pain
- How severe the pain is (Many doctors and nurses will ask you to rate the severity, for example, using a scale of 0 to 10, with 0 being no pain at all and 10 being the worst pain you can imagine.)
- What the pain feels like (e.g., sharp, achy, gnawing)
- Whether you have the pain all the time or only at certain times
- What makes it worse and what makes it better
- How it affects your ability to sleep, your appetite, your activity, your desire to be with friends and family, and your mood

Medications for treating pain are called **analgesics**. Many different analgesics are available, and they are often prescribed in a stepwise approach, starting with a mild analgesic and progressing to a stronger one as needed until your pain is controlled. First-line over-the-counter analgesics include acetaminophen, aspirin, and nonsteroidal anti-inflammatory drugs (NSAIDs) (e.g., ibuprofen, naproxen). If these medications are not effective, your doctor will prescribe an opioid or narcotic analgesic (e.g., morphine, oxycodone,

There is no benefit at all to having pain.

Comfort, Activity, and Sleep

Analgesics
Medications for treating pain.

51

hydromorphone, fentanyl). Other medications are effective in relieving pain when used in combination with analgesics: certain antidepressant, anticonvulsant, anti-inflammatory, and steroid medications.

Pain medications come in many forms: tablets, liquids to swallow, liquids to be absorbed under the tongue, skin patches, and rectal suppositories. Also, solutions can be given intravenously (into the vein) via a portable pump. The pump is often set to deliver a steady dose of medication into the bloodstream with extra doses that you can deliver as needed. The pump is set up to allow so-called patient-controlled medication administration with a limit to prevent overdose.

Chronic pain medication works most effectively when given on a regular schedule around the clock. This regimen keeps a steady level of pain medication in your bloodstream to prevent you from experiencing pain.

New long-acting medications are very helpful because they last for many hours or even days. You don't need to take long-acting medication as frequently as you do the immediate-release (short-acting) forms. However, even with long-acting medication, most people require an immediate-release pain medication for what is called *break-through pain*. This is pain or discomfort that you experience during the day or night despite taking the long-acting medication.

When using the immediate-release pain medication, take it as frequently as you need to based on the instructions on the bottle. If you wait too long between doses and the pain becomes severe, the medication will not work as quickly or as effectively. If you find you need the immediate-release pain medication frequently during the day or that it is not effective, ask your doctor about increasing the dose of the long-acting medication.

Of all the many different types of pain medication, what works for one person may not work as well for another. Finding the right medication and the right dose and schedule to keep you without pain might take some time. Be persistent in working with your doctor and nurse until you find a regimen that works for you. If you do not feel satisfied with the degree of relief you are getting, ask the doctor about a referral to a pain specialist. You can also find a pain specialist by calling the Cancer Information Service of the National Cancer Institute or the American Cancer Society.

Finding the right medication and the right dose and schedule to keep you without pain might take some time.

Some people are concerned about taking pain medication because they are afraid that, if they take it for milder pain, it won't work if they need it later for severe pain. Many pain medications, particularly narcotics, have no maximal dose. In other words, the dose can be increased indefinitely over time, so that you can be sure to get good pain relief if you need it at some point in the future, no matter how severe your pain may be.

There are several reasons to call your doctor about pain:
- **You are not getting adequate pain relief from your medication.**
- **On a scale of 0 to 10, with 0 being no pain and 10 being the worst pain you can imagine, your pain is at a level of 5 or higher most of the time.**
- **You are not able to sleep because of pain.**
- **You are not taking the full dose of pain medicine because of its side effects.**

Comfort, Activity, and Sleep

For more information on how to manage pain, the National Cancer Institute has a booklet entitled *Pain Control: A Guide for People with Cancer and Their Families.* This is available on the Internet (www.cancer.gov/cancerinfo/paincontrol), or you can order it over the phone by calling the Cancer Information Service at 800-4-CANCER. For more information, search on these other Internet sites:

- *Cancer-Pain.org:* www.cancer-pain.org
- *American Cancer Society:* www.cancer.org
- *Oncology Nursing Society:* www.cancersymptoms.org
- *American Society of Clinical Oncology:* www.cancer.net

26. What can I do about the side effects I get from my pain medication?

Pete's comment:

My pain medication, like most, had a side effect of constipation. This was managed by a combination of Colace and Senokot. I also included prunes in my diet and drank plenty of fluids. After several weeks, constipation was no longer a problem and I was able to eliminate the medication.

Some people are concerned about taking pain medication because of the side effects. Common side effects from pain medication are sleepiness, nausea, and constipation.

- Sleepiness generally passes after a few days. However, if the sleepiness persists, ask your doctor or nurse about adjusting the dose or adding another medication to counteract it.
- Nausea also commonly passes after a few days on pain medication. If it does not, ask your doctor

about trying a different pain medication or about taking medication to relieve the nausea.

- Unfortunately, constipation from pain medications does not pass. Taking a combination of a stool softener (e.g., docusate) and a laxative (e.g., senna, bisacodyl, lactulose, polyethylene glycol) on a regular basis can help. Newer medications may be more helpful for some patients on high doses of narcotics for a long time. These are MiraLAX (polyethylene glycol), a powder taken mixed in water, and Relistor (methylnaltrexone bromide), an injection. Ask your doctor or nurse about which medications you should take for constipation, what dose, and how often you should take them. Increasing the amount of liquid you drink during the day will also help reduce the likelihood of constipation.

If you become dizzy or confused from the pain medication, tell your doctor or nurse. Switching the dose or type of medication will usually resolve this problem.

27. I am afraid of taking my pain medication because I don't want to get addicted. What should I do?

Some people are concerned about taking pain medication because they are afraid of becoming addicted. Pain medication does not cause addiction when it is taken to treat pain. However, when taken on a regular basis, it does cause *tolerance*, that is, your body physically adjusts to the level of medication in your bloodstream. If you stop the medication suddenly, you can develop withdrawal symptoms. To prevent these symptoms, if you no longer need your pain medication, taper down the dose of medication gradually rather than stopping it suddenly. Your doctor or nurse will

Pain medication does not cause addiction when it is taken to treat pain.

Comfort, Activity, and Sleep

review with you exactly how to do this. Tolerance to the medication is not **addiction**, which is a desire or craving for the medication to feel high rather than to have your pain relieved. Research studies show that it is extremely rare for patients with cancer to develop addiction from pain medication.

Addiction

A desire or craving for the medication to feel high rather than to have your pain relieved.

28. Are there other treatments for pain that do not rely on taking medication?

For some types of pain, surgery may be helpful by removing all or part of the tumor causing the pain. However, surgery is not an option for many people; in that case, other treatments may be offered.

Radiation therapy is effective in treating some types of cancer pain. With external beam radiation therapy, a beam of energy is directed from a treatment machine at precise angles toward a defined target in your body. The therapy can reduce pain by shrinking a tumor that is pressing on or invading surrounding organs or nerves. If you do not feel your pain is controlled adequately with your medication, ask your doctor if radiation therapy would be helpful. However, if your cancer has spread widely throughout your body, external beam radiation is unlikely to be effective for you.

For people who have bone metastasis (spread of the primary tumor to the bone) in multiple areas of the body, treatment with a radioactive isotope may be helpful. Strontium-89 is injected into the blood, travels through the body, and collects in the bone where the tumors have spread. It then emits radiation to those areas to shrink the tumors, thus reducing the pain.

If pain is caused by pressure on a nerve, a procedure called a **nerve block** can sometimes be performed. This involves injecting a local anesthetic or alcohol into or around the nerve near the point where the tumor is pressing. The injected substance blocks the transmission of messages from the nerve to the brain, so that you are no longer aware of the pressure. Blocks may also be done surgically; that is, the nerves are cut to relieve the pain. If you do not feel your pain is controlled adequately with your current medication, ask your doctor if this would be helpful.

A variety of nonmedical strategies may be helpful in treating pain, either alone or in combination with your pain medication: distraction, relaxation, imagery, prayer, meditation, and acupuncture. Specialists in these techniques can perform them or train you to use them to control your pain. If you are interested in them, ask your doctor or nurse for a referral, or contact the National Center for Complementary and Alternative Medicine.

29. What can I do for flu-like symptoms?

Flu-like symptoms may be caused by infection, cancer, or treatment for cancer. These symptoms are most commonly fever, chills, aches and pains in the muscles (**myalgias**), and fatigue. You might also experience decreased appetite, headache, nausea, vomiting, or diarrhea.

If you develop these symptoms, call your doctor or nurse. Always immediately report fever of 100.5°F or greater, with or without chills, to your doctor's office unless the fever is a known chronic problem. If these symptoms are new, you need to make sure you don't

Nerve block

Injecting a local anesthetic or alcohol into or around the nerve near the point where the tumor is pressing.

Myalgias

Aches and pains in the muscles.

Comfort, Activity, and Sleep

have an infection. The doctor will ask you questions, perform a physical examination, take blood samples, and perhaps perform other tests. If you have an infection, treatment will be prescribed.

When a cancer causes flu-like symptoms, they are commonly referred to as *tumor fever*. Many people with tumor fever experience symptoms on a daily basis and usually at the same time (or times) each day. Very often, when treatment of the cancer results in remission or cure, tumor fever goes away.

Certain treatments for cancer can cause flu-like symptoms. If these symptoms are likely to occur from your treatment or from other medications, your doctor or nurse will tell you. The reaction can occur while you are receiving the medication, within a few hours, or even several days after the treatment. Flu-like symptoms can be caused by:

- Chemotherapy, such as gemcitabine, dacarbazine, and bleomycin.
- Biologic therapy (therapy that boosts your immune system to fight the cancer), such as interferon or interleukin, and monoclonal antibodies, such as rituximab and trastuzumab.
- Medicines to strengthen bone, such as pamidronate and zoledronic acid.

If you are likely to experience these symptoms while you are receiving the medication, the doctor or nurse will give you premedication (before the treatment) to prevent the reaction: acetaminophen, diphenhydramine, nonsteroidal anti-inflammatory medication (ibuprofen, naproxen), or even meperidine or morphine.

If you experience flu-like symptoms at home, regardless of the reason, the following measures may help:

- Your doctor may prescribe acetaminophen or non-steroidal anti-inflammatory medicines (e.g., naproxen) for you to take around the clock (on a regular basis).
- Drink plenty of fluids to prevent dehydration from fever.
- Take cool to tepid sponge baths to keep your fever down.
- Take regular uninterrupted rest periods if you are tired.
- Ask your doctor to prescribe medicine for nausea, vomiting, and diarrhea if you develop these (see Questions 55 to 57 for more information).

30. What can I do to treat itching?

Itching is a sensation that makes people want to scratch. The medical term for this is **pruritus**. Itchiness can occur on one area of the body (*localized*), or it can affect the entire body (*generalized*). It may also be accompanied by a rash or other skin changes. In patients with cancer, itching can have a number of causes:

- Some cancers, including leukemia, lymphoma, and cancers of the stomach, lung, or breast, may be associated with itching.
- Some chemotherapy medicines may cause itching, such as doxorubicin and erlotinib.
- Radiation therapy may cause skin changes, including itching. If you are being treated with radiation, contact your doctor or nurse before applying anything new to your skin to soothe irritation.
- Some medicines, including pain medicine (narcotic analgesics like morphine) and antibiotics, can cause itching.

Pruritus

A sensation that makes people want to scratch.

If you are being treated with radiation, contact your doctor or nurse before applying anything new to your skin to soothe irritation.

- An allergic reaction to medicine can cause itching.
- Other diseases, such as liver disease and kidney failure, may be associated with itching. (**Jaundice** is characterized by a yellowing of the skin and the whites of the eyes resulting from a buildup of bilirubin in the tissues; it can occur if the bile ducts are blocked or if the liver is not functioning, and is accompanied by a darkening of the urine and a lightening of stool color.)
- Other causes are dry skin, insect bites, and changes in the soap or laundry detergent.

Jaundice

Yellowing of the skin and the whites of the eyes resulting from a buildup of bilirubin in the tissues; it can occur if the bile ducts are blocked or if the liver is not functioning, and is accompanied by a darkening of the urine and a lightening of stool color.

Constant scratching can cause more irritation to the skin and, in some people, a break in the skin that can bring about additional discomfort and even infection. Itching can interfere with your sleep and overall quality of life. If you have itching, a rash, redness, or breakdown of your skin, contact your doctor or nurse before applying anything to your body. The doctor will ask you many questions, inspect your skin, and possibly take a blood sample. Be prepared to give them the following information:

- The area that is affected, when it started, and what makes it better or worse
- Medicines that you are taking, including prescription and over-the-counter medicine (Be sure to tell them about any new medicines.)
- Changes in your skin, such as rash, hives, or dryness, and changes in the color of your skin, such as redness or yellow skin (jaundice)

If the cancer is causing the itching, treatment resulting in remission or cure often stops it. If the itching is caused by a medicine, your doctor may stop the medicine or switch to another one that won't cause itching. If you have itchiness or a skin reaction from radiation treatments, speak to your nurse about specific skin recommendations for people receiving radiation therapy.

There are many treatments for itching. Here are some general measures that almost anyone can try:

- Bathe or shower using tepid water and a superfatted unscented soap (e.g., Dove). Aveeno oatmeal baths may also be soothing.
- Use emollient lotions, such as Curél or Lubriderm.
- Keep your fingernails trimmed.
- Keep the air humidified.
- Drink plenty of fluids.
- Wear loose-fitting cotton clothing; use cotton sheets.
- Apply cool compresses for localized itching.
- Use distraction measures, relaxation techniques, or guided visual imagery.

Your doctor or nurse might suggest other treatments:

- Steroid creams, either by prescription or over-the-counter;
- Topical or oral antihistamines (e.g., diphenhydramine);
- Sedatives for those who are unable to sleep;
- Referral to a dermatologist for a consultation.

Lisa's comment:

Pruritis associated with the radiation field drove me crazy. Even though I used all recommended creams (Biafine, Bactroban Ointment, Betamethasone Dipropionate Ointment), I still found myself scratching absentmindedly. I felt that I needed to put myself in mittens, in addition to keeping my fingernails short, in order to prevent significant skin breakdown.

Comfort, Activity, and Sleep

ACTIVITY AND SLEEP

31. I feel tired much of the time. What can I do to increase my energy?

Lisa's comment:

I am a single professional woman. I have elderly parents who live across town, a brother who lives 15 miles away, and numerous friends who live both near and far. I am an independent individual. I insisted on getting myself to and from my treatments (chemotherapy) via mass transportation, alone—I live about 30 miles from the Cancer Center. My fatigue was significant, but generally occurred a few days after treatment. My parents and friends wanted to drive me to my treatments, but I wouldn't allow them. My mother, therefore, took on the added chore of doing my laundry and food shopping every week. My parents' help significantly contributed to my increased energy levels. It allowed me to save my energy for long workdays.

Mary Ann's comment:

I wish I had the magic answer as to what to do about the fatigue that accompanies my treatment. I, too, am tired all the time. I was doing a whole lot of napping but have now tried pushing through that 3 o'clock (or 10 a.m., 11 a.m., 2 p.m., 4 p.m., 6 p.m.—anytime) exhaustion. Sometimes it works, sometimes it doesn't. Caffeine is not the answer and I find myself drinking Gatorade of all things! I always thought of it as some fancy Kool-Aid but have discovered, thanks to the advice of my oncologist, that it does add something back to your system. It really has helped me (and it comes in a low-calorie variety but good luck finding it!)

Fatigue is a common problem for people with cancer. You may feel tired, weak, or weary; lack energy; be unable to concentrate; or feel irritable or depressed. Many things may cause fatigue:

- The disease itself
- The treatment you are receiving
- The side effects of certain medications (e.g., medications to treat pain or nausea)
- **Anemia** (a low red blood cell count)
- A decrease in the amount of food you eat
- A decrease in the amount of liquids you drink
- Difficulty sleeping
- Emotional distress
- Chronic pain

Anemia

A low red blood cell count.

However, many people with cancer develop fatigue without any clear single cause.

Sleeping extra hours at night, by going to bed earlier or staying in bed a bit later in the morning, will improve your energy. Resting during the day is also important: napping for short periods or just lying down and relaxing. Plan these rest periods for times when you know you will be more likely to feel tired. Even bathing, dressing, or eating may cause some people to feel tired, and they should plan time for a short rest after these activities. However, at the same time, you want to push yourself to be as active as possible. Lying in bed all day generally makes you weaker. In fact, there is evidence that exercising will actually increase your energy level as long as you don't push yourself to the point of exhaustion. If you are currently exercising on a regular basis, try to maintain your schedule, adjusting the intensity and frequency of your exercise regimen according to how you feel. If you are not currently exercising, take a daily walk. Start with 5 to 15 minutes a day. Adjust the distance and pace

Comfort, Activity, and Sleep

*The key thing
is to find a
balance
between rest
and activity.*

based on how you feel. The key thing is to find a balance between rest and activity.

Anemia, one cause of fatigue, may be treated with a medication called epoetin (Procrit, Epogen) or darbepoetin (Aranesp). This medication stimulates your bone marrow to make more red blood cells, raising your blood cell count and increasing your energy. It is given by injection under the skin using a very small thin needle. It comes in different doses and is commonly given once a week. You may be instructed to take an iron supplement by mouth while getting these injections. If you are anemic and feel fatigued, ask your doctor if this medication could help you.

If you have other specific problems that you think may be contributing to your fatigue, speak with your doctor or nurse about them. Ask them about taking a sleeping medication if you are having difficulty sleeping at night. Ask them about how to manage your pain better if you are not comfortable. Ask about how you can cope with emotional distress better. Ask them for advice on how to increase your food and fluid intake if you feel you are not eating and drinking enough. Unfortunately, fatigue cannot always be effectively treated. It is often necessary to adjust your activity to accommodate to changes in your energy level.

Conserve your energy for the most important activities. Think about all the things you do during the day: working, shopping, cooking, cleaning, household chores, errands, taking care of children or dependent relatives, being with family and friends, and recreational or leisure activities. Which of these activities are the most important? Which give you the most pleasure? Which make you feel good about yourself? Save your energy for them.

You'll probably notice that your energy is greater at certain times of the day. Plan your favorite activities for those times. For the other things that must get done, ask family and friends to help. People often want to be helpful but don't know how. Tell them specifically what you need help with; they will probably be grateful for the direction. See Question 96 for suggestions on how family and friends can help.

Finally, let go of the things you don't need to do and don't want to do.

To learn more about fatigue, search on the following Internet sites:

- *Oncology Nursing Society:* www.cancersymptoms.org
- *American Society of Clinical Oncology:* www.cancer. net
- *National Cancer Institute:* www.cancer.gov
- *American Cancer Society:* www.cancer.org

32. I have difficulty sleeping at night. What can I do to sleep better and feel more rested?

Difficulty sleeping is a common problem for many people—either with falling asleep in the evening or with staying asleep through the night. Aside from the distress of lying awake in bed for many hours, not getting enough sleep may cause you to feel irritable and tired during the day and to have difficulty concentrating.

Try to determine whether there is a concrete reason you are not sleeping. Are you physically uncomfortable or in pain? Are you having other symptoms, like nausea, vomiting, diarrhea, constipation, itching, mouth sores, or anything else that is preventing sleep? Take medication,

Try to determine whether there is a concrete reason you are not sleeping.

as prescribed, to get a restful night's sleep. If you are taking medication and it is not effective, tell your doctor or nurse.

Aside from physical reasons for not sleeping, are you feeling anxious and worried at night? Are your thoughts racing and keeping you awake at night? Speak with someone you trust, someone supportive, about your thoughts and feelings; this may provide a significant amount of relief. Also see Questions 88 to 89, which describe the emotional reactions that people with cancer may experience and which suggest ways of feeling more in control. For some people, medication for anxiety may be helpful.

Do you feel generally restless at night, unable to relax and sleep? A variety of techniques may help:

- Establish a regular schedule, going to bed and waking up at the same times every day.
- Even if you do not sleep well at night, try not to sleep excessively during the day. Naps disrupt your body's normal cycle. If you are very tired, take a short nap during the day, but not for more than an hour.
- Avoid being in bed at any time except when you are going to sleep. When resting during the day, lay in another room, on a couch or chair. Use your bed only for sleep at night.
- Avoid drinking caffeine or stimulants after dinner.

For some people, these techniques aren't helpful. If you continue to have difficulty with sleep, ask your doctor to prescribe a sleeping medication. Getting a restful sleep at night is important to feeling energized and capable during the day.

33. Is there medication I can take to treat my fatigue?

One cause of fatigue is anemia, a low red blood cell count. Red blood cells are produced in the bone marrow and released into the bloodstream, where they carry oxygen from the lungs to all the tissues of the body. The cells use the oxygen to create energy. When the red blood cell count is low, less oxygen is available to the cells, resulting in fatigue.

The number of cells in the blood can be measured by testing a blood sample for what is called a *complete blood count* (*CBC*). The number of red cells is also reflected in measurements called **hematocrit** (the percentage of red cells in the blood) and **hemoglobin** (the substance in red blood cells that binds to oxygen and carries it to the tissues of the body). The normal ranges for these tests vary from laboratory to laboratory, but in general they are as follows:

- Hemoglobin: 12–18 grams per deciliter (g/dl)
- Hematocrit: 36–54%

Of the many causes of fatigue (see Question 31), if the cause is anemia, your doctor will need to determine the reason for it and decide how to treat it. If you are undergoing chemotherapy and your hemoglobin is lower than 10 g/dl, treatment with a medication called epoetin (Procrit, Epogen) or darbepoetin (Aranesp) may be helpful. This medication stimulates your bone marrow to make more red blood cells, raising your blood cell count, delivering more oxygen to the body, and increasing your energy. It is given by injection under the skin using a very small thin needle. It comes in different doses and is commonly given once a week. Your doctor may also decide to treat your anemia with

Comfort, Activity, and Sleep

Hematocrit

The percentage of red cells in the blood.

Hemoglobin

The substance in red blood cells that binds to oxygen and carries it to the tissues of the body.

a blood transfusion. Both treatments have their risks and benefits, and you and your doctor will decide which is best for you. Along with either treatment, you may also be instructed to take an iron supplement. You can obtain additional information about the use of epoetin and darbepoetin on the Internet (www.cancer. net/ patient/Publications+and+Resources/What+to+ Know%3A+ASCO's+Guidelines/What+to+Know %3A +ASCO's+Guideline+on+Epoetin+and+Darbepoetin+ Treatment).

34. Can I exercise?

Pete's comment:

Exercise has been an integral part of my life for the last 20 years, and I was concerned that my cancer treatment might cause me to cut back. I was encouraged by my oncology team to ease back into an exercise regimen as quickly as possible. I started with chair aerobics and one-on-one personal training with a clinical nurse specialist. I was eventually able to get back to a full workout routine at my gym, which has given me both a mental and physical lift.

The benefits of exercise are well-known. The American Cancer Society and other organizations recommend exercise for promoting health and for the prevention of many diseases (e.g., heart disease, high blood pressure, cancer). Many studies have shown that exercise may play a role in the prevention of breast, prostate, and colon cancers.

Some people believe that they should "conserve their energy" during the diagnosis, treatment, and recovery phases of cancer. However, having a diagnosis of cancer does not mean you have to stop exercising. Studies have shown that people with cancer enjoy many benefits from exercise, including:

People with cancer enjoy many benefits from exercise.

- Reduced feelings of anxiety, stress, and depression
- Decreased treatment-related side effects (nausea, constipation, and fatigue)
- Improved appetite and sleep
- Improved bone strength and muscular flexibility
- Improved quality of life and feelings of general well-being

Here are some general guidelines about exercise:

- Before you start or resume exercising, check with your doctor or nurse to see whether you should avoid some types of activity.
- Most people have no limitations on exercise. If exercise was a part of your routine before cancer diagnosis, you should be able to keep up the same routine during diagnosis and treatment.
- After some types of surgery (breast surgery, lung surgery), your doctor or nurse will recommend therapeutic exercises.
- Exercise should not cause pain or discomfort. You should participate in enjoyable activities.

If you have been in bed or have not exercised in a long time, performing everyday activities yourself is a good way to get started. Adding exercise to your daily routine can be as simple as taking a walk outside to get the paper or mail, doing light housekeeping, or shopping for food. In general, it is important to start slowly and increase your exercise level gradually.

Others may enjoy yoga or other structured exercise classes offered at fitness centers. Exercise and yoga videotapes are also available at public libraries for those who want to work out at home. Some people participate in aerobic exercise and weight-training activities.

If exercise was a part of your routine before cancer diagnosis, you should be able to keep up the same routine during diagnosis and treatment.

Comfort, Activity, and Sleep

Studies have shown that structured exercise programs helped cancer patients improve endurance, strength, and flexibility, and these patients return to everyday activity faster than those who do not exercise.

There may be specific exercise groups in your area for cancer survivors or those who are actively undergoing cancer treatment. Your local chapter of the American Cancer Society may be able to direct you to such a program. Additionally, some hospitals and universities have wellness programs (including nutrition and exercise) for people with cancer. Local fitness centers (e.g., the YMCA) may also provide classes for those undergoing cancer treatments.

PART FOUR

Blood Counts and Skin Problems

I have heard that chemotherapy may cause drops in my blood counts. What does this mean?

What do I do if my red blood cell count is low?

What is shingles? Is there is a vaccine for shingles, and should I get it?

More . . .

BLOOD COUNTS AND YOUR IMMUNE SYSTEM

35. I have heard that chemotherapy may cause drops in my blood counts. What does this mean?

Bone marrow produces blood cells and releases them into the bloodstream, where they are able to protect the body in a variety of ways.

White blood cells

Cells in the blood that fight off infection and other types of disease; there are many different types of white blood cells, including neutrophils and lymphocytes; also called leukocytes.

Platelets

Cells in the blood that stop bleeding by clumping together, or clotting, to plug up damaged blood vessels; also called thrombocytes.

Red blood cells

Cells in the blood that contain hemoglobin that carries oxygen from the lungs to all the tissues in the body, which the cells use to create energy; also called erythrocytes.

- **White blood cells** are cells in the blood that fight off infection and other types of disease; there are many different types of white blood cells, including neutrophils and lymphocytes.
- If you are cut or injured, **platelets**, also called *thrombocytes*, are blood cells that stop bleeding by clumping together, or clotting, to plug up damaged blood vessels.
- **Red blood cells**, also called erythrocytes, are cells in the blood that contain hemoglobin that carries oxygen from the lungs to all the tissues in the body; the cells use the oxygen to create energy.

The number of cells in the blood can be measured by testing a blood sample for a complete blood count (CBC). The number of red cells is also reflected in measurements called *hematocrit* (the percentage of red cells in the blood) and *hemoglobin* (the amount of the molecule carrying the oxygen in the red cells). The normal ranges for a CBC vary from laboratory to laboratory, but in general the normal values are as follows:

- *White blood cells:* 4–10,000 cells per cubic millimeter (cells/mm^3)
- *Platelets:* 150,000–500,000 cells/mm^3

- *Hemoglobin:* 12–18 g/dl
- *Hematocrit:* 36–54%

Once the bone marrow releases the blood cells into the bloodstream, they live for only a short time: as short as 24 hours for some types of white cells, about 10 days for platelets, and about 3 months for red cells. The body depends on the rapidly dividing cells in the bone marrow to continuously replace these cells as they die.

Chemotherapy destroys tumor cells by preventing them from dividing. However, normal cells that divide rapidly, such as those in the bone marrow, are also very sensitive to chemotherapy. The bone marrow loses the ability to form new blood cells; so fewer cells are released into the bloodstream, and the blood counts drop, generally 7 to 14 days after a chemotherapy treatment. The white cells and platelets are particularly sensitive because they live only a short period of time.

The body can adjust to slight decreases in the number of blood cells without any problem; however, your doctor will order a CBC before you get each cycle of chemotherapy to be sure that your counts are not too low. If your white cell or platelet count is too low, your doctor may decide to hold your treatment for a week to give the bone marrow a chance to make new blood cells. See Questions 36 and 37 for other measures that may be taken if your blood counts are low.

Radiation therapy may also cause a drop in your blood cell counts if it is directed to an area that contains a large amount of active bone marrow, such as the pelvis, the ribs, or the spinal column. If there is a chance that your blood cell counts will drop during treatment, your doctor will order a CBC every week or two during your treatment.

Blood Counts and Skin Problems

36. What do I do if my white blood cell count is low?

If your white blood cell (WBC) count drops, the question is which types of white blood cells are low? The doctor will order a CBC that lists the different types of white blood cells found and the number of each. **Neutrophils**, a type of white blood cell that fights bacterial infection and other diseases, make up about 45–75% of your white blood cells. If the count is low, you have an increased risk of developing an infection.

Throughout your treatment, you can do certain things to prevent infection:

- Wash your hands frequently with soap and water, especially before eating and after going to the bathroom.
- Bathe daily with soap and water, and brush your teeth after each meal.
- Avoid people with colds or flu.
- Avoid sharing food utensils, drinking glasses, or toothbrushes.
- Avoid handling pet feces or urine, especially in cat litter or birdcage droppings.
- Check with your doctor or nurse before having any dental work or immunizations.

You can develop **neutropenia,** a decrease in the number of neutrophils, the type of white blood cell that fights bacterial infection and other diseases. In that event, your doctor or nurse may advise you to take extra precautions to prevent infection. In addition, your doctor may prescribe a medication called filgrastim (Neupogen®) or pegfilgrastim (Neulasta®) that can stimulate the bone marrow to make new white cells quickly. It is injected under your skin with a small

Neutrophils

A type of white blood cell that fights infection and other diseases.

Neutropenia

A decrease in the number of neutrophils, the type of white blood cell that fights bacterial infection and other diseases.

Your doctor or nurse may advise you to take extra precautions to prevent infection.

thin needle. You or a family member may be taught to give the injection at home.

Despite doing all the right things, you may still develop an infection. If you have any implanted catheters or tubes (such as a port, a urinary stent, or a biliary stent) you have a higher than normal risk of developing an infection. You will not feel that your WBC count is low, so call your doctor or nurse if you develop any signs or symptoms of infection. You will most likely need to be examined and have tests taken to determine whether you require treatment with antibiotics.

Reasons to call the doctor:
- **Fever of 100.5°F (38°C) or higher**
- **Shaking chills**
- **Sore throat or cough**
- **Frequency or burning when you urinate**
- **Swelling, redness, or pain anywhere on your skin**
- **Vomiting or diarrhea unrelated to your chemotherapy**

To learn more about neutropenia and how to manage it, search on the following Internet sites:

- *Oncology Nursing Society:* www.cancersymptoms.org
- *American Society of Clinical Oncology:* www.cancer.net
- *National Cancer Institute:* www.cancer.gov
- *American Cancer Society:* www.cancer.org

37. What do I do if my platelet count is low?

If your platelet count drops, there is an increased risk of bleeding. Throughout your treatment, unless prescribed by your doctor, avoid aspirin, products that contain aspirin, and nonsteroidal anti-inflammatory drugs (NSAIDs), such as ibuprofen, because these may all interfere with platelet functioning. If the platelet

If your platelet count drops, there is an increased risk of bleeding.

count drops very low, your doctor or nurse may advise you to take extra precautions to prevent bleeding, such as using only an electric razor and avoiding activities in which you could be injured.

You will not feel that your platelet count is low; so call your doctor or nurse if you develop any signs or symptoms of bleeding.

Reasons to call the doctor:
• **Easy bruising**
• **Bleeding gums or nosebleeds**
• **Blood in the urine or stool**
• **Black stools**

38. What do I do if my red blood cell count is low?

If the red blood cell (RBC) count drops, you will feel fatigued. Fatigue can be experienced in many different ways: lacking energy; feeling tired, weak, or weary; feeling irritable or depressed; or having difficulty concentrating. You may even feel lightheaded or short of breath. For suggestions on how to conserve energy and manage fatigue, see Question 31.

If the RBC count falls very low, your doctor may recommend a medication called epoetin (Procrit®, Epogen®) or darbepoetin (Aranesp®), which stimulates the bone marrow to make more red blood cells. It is given by injection under the skin using a very small thin needle. It comes in different doses and can be given either three times a week or once every 1 to 2 weeks. Some people give themselves the injection; some people get it from their oncology nurse. You may also be instructed to take an iron supplement by mouth while getting these injections.

To learn more about anemia and how to manage fatigue, search on the following Internet sites:

- *Oncology Nursing Society:* www.cancersymptoms.org
- *American Society of Clinical Oncology:* www.cancer.net
- *National Cancer Institute:* www.cancer.gov
- *American Cancer Society*: www.cancer.org

CARING FOR YOUR SKIN AND HAIR

39. I have heard that radiation therapy causes a skin reaction. Is this true? How should I care for my skin during radiation therapy?

Radiation therapy is administered as a beam of energy directed from a treatment machine at precise angles toward a defined target in your body. It destroys tumor cells in its path by preventing them from dividing. Normal cells that divide rapidly are also very sensitive to radiation therapy. As a result, there may be changes in your skin where the beam enters and exits your body. After about 2 weeks, you may notice redness, tanning, dryness, flaking, and/or itching. If you are being treated in sensitive areas of the body, such as the armpit, the neck, under the breasts, and the perineum (the area between the genitals and the anus), the reactions may become more severe over time, and you may develop blistering and weeping of the skin. Ask your doctor or nurse to explain what you should expect based on the area being treated. These effects are all expected, and they will heal about a month after treatment is completed; however, you may be left with an area of darkened skin in the treated area.

Blood Counts and Skin Problems

Take special care of your skin from the first day of treatment.

Take special care of your skin from the first day of treatment to ensure that you do not become uncomfortable from any changes. Bathe daily using warm water and a mild, unscented soap, such as Dove, Neutrogena, Basis, or Cetaphil. Do not scrub the skin with a cloth or brush, rinse the skin well to get off all the soap, and gently pat it dry. Your doctor or nurse may recommend the use of a moisturizer, either from the beginning of treatment or if you develop dryness or itching. Examples of products often used during radiation therapy are Aquaphor, Eucerin, Biafine Topical Emulsion, and products with aloe vera gel, calendula, or hyaluronic acid. There is no compelling evidence that any one product is better than the other. Ask your doctor or nurse for a recommendation on application. The common recommendation is to use the moisturizer twice a day, after your daily treatment and at bedtime. Check before using any other lotions, creams, or ointments in the area being treated because some products can make the skin reaction more severe.

Avoid irritating the skin. Follow these suggestions in the area being treated:

- Avoid tight, constricting clothing.
- If treatment is to the pelvis, wear cotton underwear.
- Avoid the use of tape.
- Avoid scratching the skin. Tell your doctor or nurse if the moisturizers are not effective in relieving the itching so that something else can be prescribed.
- Avoid direct sunlight.
- Avoid the use of ice packs or heating pads.

Radiation therapy will also cause the hair in the treated area to fall out. If you are not being treated in the head or neck area, you will not lose any hair on your head. Your hair will grow back several months after your treatment is completed.

40. I have heard that chemotherapy may cause me to lose my hair. Can I prevent this? What can I do to feel good about my appearance if I lose my hair?

Chemotherapy destroys tumor cells by preventing them from dividing, and normal cells that divide rapidly are also very sensitive to chemotherapy. The cells at the base of the hair follicle may become unable to divide to make new cells, weakening the hair shaft and resulting in hair loss. Some people experience only a thinning of their hair, but others lose all the hair on their head. Certain chemotherapy drugs are much more likely than others to cause hair loss. Your doctor or nurse can tell you if you are likely to lose your hair based on the type of chemotherapy drug that you are receiving.

Certain chemotherapy drugs are much more likely than others to cause hair loss.

If you are receiving chemotherapy drugs that are likely to cause hair loss, you might lose hair from other parts of your body. Hair anywhere on your body can be affected, including your eyebrows, eyelashes, and hair in your underarm and pubic areas. Hair loss usually begins about 3 weeks after chemotherapy begins. Sometimes people notice a gradual thinning and loss of hair, but with some chemotherapy agents the hair can come out in clumps over a period of only a few days.

If you are receiving chemotherapy that causes only a thinning of hair, you can reduce the amount of hair you lose:

- Use a mild shampoo, such as baby shampoo.
- Use a soft-bristled hairbrush.

Blood Counts and Skin Problems

- Avoid permanents and hair dyes.
- Avoid heated rollers and high-heat hair dryers.

If you are receiving chemotherapy with a high likelihood of causing complete hair loss, there is no way of preventing this. Doctors no longer use ice caps to prevent the chemotherapy from flowing to the scalp because they want to be sure the chemotherapy travels all over your body, not missing any area where there could be cancer cells.

If you are likely to lose your hair from treatment, you may find it helpful to purchase a wig or hairpiece beforehand. Some people like to match their own hairstyle to maintain their usual appearance; others like to try a new look. Wigs can be made with human hair or from synthetic fibers, and they vary considerably in price. Look for stores in your area that specialize in working with people who lose their hair from cancer treatment, or you can purchase a wig or hairpiece through the American Cancer Society. Your local American Cancer Society or hospital social work department may also have wigs and hairpieces available on loan. Your insurance company may cover the cost of the hairpiece. Check your policy, and, if it is covered, ask your doctor to write you a prescription for a "hair prosthesis needed for cancer treatment." Costs that are not reimbursed are tax deductible.

Do whatever makes you feel most comfortable.

Some people prefer to wear a turban, scarf, or cap to cover their heads, and some prefer to leave their head uncovered. Do whatever makes you feel the most comfortable. The important thing is not to let your changed appearance alter your willingness to interact with family, friends, and coworkers. Despite the loss of hair, you can take many steps to feel good about your appearance: for example, taking care in the clothes you wear, using makeup if you like, and wearing scarves or caps. The Personal Care Products Council, the National Cosmetology Association, and the American Cancer Society sponsor a free program, "Look Good, Feel Better," that is dedicated to helping men and women being treated for cancer feel better about their appearance. The program offers beauty techniques that help restore your appearance and enhance your self-image, provides many tips on its Internet site, and presents group programs all over the country. To find out if the program is available in your area, check their Internet site (www. lookgoodfeelbetter.org) or call 800-395-LOOK.

41. I have heard there may be changes in the color of my skin from my treatment. What does this mean?

Color changes in skin and nails can occur during treatment for cancer. These color changes are usually temporary and can be caused by either chemotherapy or radiation therapy. Changes in skin and nails include:

Skin and nail color changes are usually temporary.

- Flushing
- Hyperpigmentation
- Photosensitivity

Flushing is a temporary redness that usually occurs in the face and neck as a result of dilated capillaries, which are small blood vessels located just under the surface of the skin. Flushing can be caused by chemotherapy (paclitaxel, cisplatin, doxorubicin), intravenous contrast (used with CTs), or some oral medications (steroid medicines such as prednisone or dexamethasone). Sometimes flushing is accompanied by a feeling of warmth. Flushing is always temporary and generally lasts for minutes or up to several hours.

> **Call your doctor or nurse if the flushing is persist-
> ent or accompanied by pain, fever (100.5°F or
> more), swelling, or other discomfort.**

Hyperpigmentation is a darkening of the skin, such as a
freckle. This darkening can be generalized, as in a sun-
tan, or localized to certain areas of the body. If localized,
you may notice darkening of the skin over finger joints
or elbows and knees. The palms of the hands and soles of
the feet may also darken, as may the tissue under the fingernails and toenails or the nails themselves. There may
even be color changes in your mouth, for example, darkening of your tongue and gums. Certain intravenous
chemotherapy (fluorouracil) causes darkening along the
length of the vein into which it is given. Hyperpigmentation may be more noticeable in people with darker skin
tones. Some types of chemotherapy (paclitaxel or docetaxel) cause white lines, called Beau's lines, to form hor-
izontally on the fingernails. Radiation therapy can cause
skin to darken in the irradiated area. Sun exposure may
increase hyperpigmentation temporarily. Hyperpigmentation usually occurs within several days to 2 to 3 weeks
after starting treatment. Sometimes the discoloration is
permanent, but usually it resolves within a few months
after treatment is completed.

Photosensitivity means that your skin is more sensitive
to the sun (i.e., ultraviolet radiation); you can burn
more easily when in the sun or you may develop a rash
from it. This reaction can occur whether you have light
or dark skin, and it may result from medications,
including certain types of chemotherapy and antibiotics. Radiation therapy can also cause the skin in the
treated area to be more sensitive to the sun. Before
going out in the sun, ask your doctor or nurse if you are
taking any medications that can cause this reaction.

Photosensitivity can result in severe sunburn, but this reaction can be prevented. When outside, even on cloudy days, wear protective clothing, including a hat, long-sleeved shirt, and long pants, and always use a sunscreen with an SPF of at least 15. At the beach, sit under an umbrella and use a sunblock such as zinc oxide. If you have had radiation therapy, see Question 39 for additional skin care tips.

If you get a bad sunburn or rash from the sun, call your doctor or nurse. They can prescribe medicines to make you more comfortable. They can also tell you which lotions or creams are best to use for the sunburn.

Lisa's comment:

I'm a beach bum—love the summer, love the beach, love the ocean. I have a cabana at Malibu Beach (Long Beach, Long Island). Photosensitivity was probably one of the biggest obstacles for me. I had to wear sunscreen (well, that wasn't new), sit under an umbrella, and not go in the ocean (that wasn't because of chemotherapy, but because of surgery restrictions). I felt like my one true pleasure was a chore, a burden. I did very well with keeping myself protected from the sun, but I really didn't entirely enjoy my days at the beach. But, chemotherapy didn't stop me from going! My fingernails turned a yellowish-orange color with the adriamycin/cytoxan therapy.

42. I have heard that some chemotherapy drugs can burn your skin. What does this mean?

Most chemotherapy drugs are given through a vein, and oncology nurses are specially trained to administer these drugs safely and accurately. Despite using the most careful technique, the drugs can sometimes leak out of the veins into the surrounding tissue and collect

Extravasation

A potential complication of intravenous chemotherapy administration that occurs when chemotherapy leaks from the vein into the surrounding tissue.

Vesicant

A type of chemotherapy that causes blistering or other local tissue damage if it leaks from a vein into the surrounding tissue.

If you feel pain or burning while your nurse is giving you treatment, say so right away.

under the skin (**extravasation**). In these cases, the vein is said to be "blown." The body reabsorbs most chemotherapy fluids with no ill effects. However, some chemotherapy drugs, call **vesicants**, can cause blistering or other local tissue damage if they leak from a vein into the surrounding tissue. Examples are cisplatin, doxorubicin, vincristine, and paclitaxel. Other chemotherapy drugs may cause irritation and inflammation if they leak under the skin but will not cause any tissue damage.

If you feel pain or burning while your nurse is giving you treatment, say so right away. If there is any indication that chemotherapy has leaked out of the vein, the nurse will stop the treatment and remove the needle. If the chemotherapy is a vesicant, the nurse may apply hot or cold compresses or inject or apply special medicine to the area. Keep an eye on the site over the next 2 weeks. Very rarely, serious reactions can develop. Call your doctor or nurse if you have pain, if the area becomes red or swollen, or if you see blisters or ulcers. The doctor will reevaluate you and refer you to a plastic surgeon if necessary.

Lisa's comment:

I wanted a mediport as soon as I heard I would need chemotherapy. I had always told my patients, "If I were to get chemo, I would get a mediport." I said it because I meant it. Being diagnosed with breast cancer and requiring an axillary node dissection meant I only had one arm available for intravenous therapy. I knew I was scheduled to receive adriamycin/paclitaxel—vesicants. So, I really wanted a mediport. I guess deep down I didn't trust anyone to give me chemotherapy. Needless to say, the Breast Service didn't recommend port placement for only eight cycles of chemotherapy—not worth the surgical risks. I did fine. The nurses did not have trouble with my veins, and I never had an extravasation.

43. What is jaundice and how can it be treated?

When the liver breaks down hemoglobin, the oxygen-carrying substance in red blood cells, it produces bilirubin, which is then incorporated into the bile, giving it a yellow-green color. Bile is stored in the gallbladder. After someone eats, the gallbladder pushes the bile out through the bile duct into the intestine where it digests certain types of food. The bile is then eliminated in the stool, and the bilirubin helps to give stool its usual brown color.

If bilirubin builds up in the bloodstream, it lodges in the skin and eyes, causing them to become yellow. This condition is referred to as *jaundice* (or *icterus*). Some of this excess bilirubin, as it is eliminated in the urine, darkens the urine. If the bilirubin is not able to pass into the intestine, the stools become lighter in color.

People with cancer may develop increased bilirubin and jaundice for a number of reasons. The body is either not eliminating enough bilirubin or producing too much of it. A mass in the bile duct or in the area around the duct (e.g., in the gallbladder, liver, or pancreas) may block the flow of bile though the duct, interfering with elimination. Disease in the liver may also reduce the body's ability to eliminate bilirubin. Certain blood disorders in which a large number of red blood cells are destroyed may cause increased levels of bilirubin.

Sometimes jaundice can be treated. If the bile duct is locally blocked, a small hollow tube can be inserted to open the duct by relieving the obstruction. If the liver disease or blood disorder is treatable, the bilirubin level will come down. However, if the jaundice cannot be treated, there are ways to ensure that you are comfortable.

Jaundice itself causes no pain, but the skin may become very dry and itchy. Scratching may create breaks in the skin, which could become infected; so preventing itching is important. Treating the dryness eases the itching. When bathing, avoid very hot water and use only mild soaps. Apply skin lotions or creams after bathing and throughout the day as needed to moisturize the skin. If you still feel itchy, ask your doctor for a prescription for medication to reduce the itching. See Question 30 for additional tips on how to control itching.

44. What do I do if I get a rash?

A *rash* is a skin reaction that may be *localized* to one area of the body or that may cover most or all of the body (*generalized*). Rashes may cause itching or pain.

Medicine is the most common cause of rashes, which can be a side effect of the medicine (e.g., causing an acne-like rash) or a sign of an allergic reaction. An illness caused by a virus, such as measles or shingles, can also cause rashes. Other causes are changes in laundry detergent, moisturizer, or soap.

> **If you develop a rash, call your doctor or nurse. Be prepared to tell:**
> - **Where the rash is located**
> - **What the rash looks like**
> - **When it started**
> - **Whether you have any other symptoms, such as fever, itching, or pain**

> • **If you have recently started using a new medicine**
>
> **Words that can be used to describe a rash are raised (bumpy), flat, or blistered. Describe the color, for example, as red, purplish, or skin color.**

If the rash is an expected side effect of the chemotherapy you are taking, your doctor or nurse will advise you on what products are best to use on your skin. If itching is associated with the rash, your doctor may prescribe an **antihistamine**, medication that is used to prevent or treat allergic reactions and that is sometimes given to treat itching caused by a rash. Diphenhydramine is an antihistamine that can be bought over the counter. Antihistamine may make you sleepy and give you a dry mouth. For an itchy rash, your doctor may also prescribe calamine lotion and/or taking a bath with Aveeno or oatmeal. If your rash seems to be from an allergic reaction to your medicine, the doctor may tell you to stop taking it. If your rash is from shingles, the physician will prescribe an antiviral medicine. See Question 45 for more information about shingles.

Antihistamine

Medication that is used to prevent or treat allergic reactions and that is sometimes given to treat itching caused by a rash.

> **If you also have hives or difficulty breathing, call your doctor and go to the nearest emergency room.**

Mary Ann's comment:

If you get a rash, call your doctor. There are excellent creams and powders to aid in the relief of rashes. When I first began my program, I had terrible rashes beneath my breasts, in any "fat roll" on my stomach, and in a rather-not-talk-about place. Antifungal medication resolved the problem within a few days. There is no reason to be uncomfortable. Speak up!

Blood Counts and Skin Problems

45. What is shingles? Is there is a vaccine for shingles, and should I get it?

Shingles (*herpes zoster*) is caused by the same virus that causes chicken pox. You can get shingles only if you have had chicken pox in the past, and about 1 in 10 people who have had chicken pox will get shingles. This infection is more common if you are 60 years of age or older and are getting treatment for cancer.

Once you have had chicken pox, the virus stays in your body and hibernates, remaining inactive, in the nerve cells along your spine. If the virus becomes active, it travels along a nerve tract on one side of your body. This can cause tingling, a burning type of pain, itching, and a blister-like rash that follows a line or band on the skin over the involved nerve. Very often, the pain and itching start 1 to 4 days before you can see the rash. If you develop a rash (not everyone does), the blisters are small and tear-shaped. Shingles can occur any-where on the body but occurs most often on the chest or back.

Shingles itself is not contagious (catching). However, if you have shingles, you can give chicken pox to someone who has not had chicken pox before. Your blisters will crust over and dry up in about 7 to 10 days. Once this happens, you are no longer contagious. Sometimes people continue to have pain even when the rash goes away. This is called **postherpetic neural-gia**, which is localized pain in the area where shingles was present.

Postherpetic neuralgia

Localized pain that occurs in the area where shingles was present.

If you think that you have shingles, call your doctor or nurse. Your doctor will prescribe an antiviral medicine (e.g., acyclovir, famciclovir). This medicine can be taken as a pill, given through a vein (intravenously), or applied as a cream (topically) on the blisters. You will need to take this medicine several times a day for 7 to 10 days, and you must take it just as the doctor tells you to.

If you develop postherpetic neuralgia, your doctor will prescribe pain medicine. This may be taken as a pill, or sometimes a cream is rubbed into the skin where the rash was located. If this medicine doesn't help your pain, follow up with your doctor.

Call your doctor if you:
- **Think you have shingles**
- **Have shingles near your eye**
- **Have a rash with a fever of 100.5°F or more**

A vaccine, called Zostavax, can now prevent shingles. The vaccine is recommended for people aged 60 or older because shingles is more common in this age group. Even if you have had shingles before, you can get the vaccine to prevent future outbreaks. Talk to your doctor to see if you should get the shingles vaccine.

PART FIVE

Problems with Breathing, Nutrition, Digestion, and Urination

How do I know if I need oxygen?

What can I do to increase my appetite and maintain my weight?

What can I do for mouth sores?

More . . .

46. I feel short of breath. What can I do to ease my breathing?

When people feel short of breath, they describe themselves as having difficulty breathing or being unable to get enough air. Some people say they feel "winded." **Dyspnea** is the medical term for shortness of breath. In people with cancer, shortness of breath can be caused by the cancer, by treatment for disease, or by something unrelated to cancer. Here are some causes of shortness of breath:

* Lung damage from cancer, radiation therapy, chemotherapy, or lung surgery
* A blood clot in the lung, which usually starts when a blood clot travels from a vein in the legs to the pulmonary artery, causing sudden shortness of breath (**pulmonary embolism**)
* Fluid buildup around the heart or lungs (called pericardial or pleural effusion)
* Lung infection
* Heart failure (called congestive heart failure)
* Asthma and emphysema (also known as chronic obstructive pulmonary disease, or COPD)
* Anemia (see Question 38)
* Stress or anxiety

The best way to relieve shortness of breath is to treat its cause. Even if the condition is not treatable or the cause is unknown, measures can be taken to help you breathe better. If you have shortness of breath, talk to your doctor or nurse, who will work with you to determine the best way to improve your breathing.

Your doctor may prescribe medicine to treat your shortness of breath: inhalers for asthma or emphysema, antibiotics for infection, epoetin for anemia, or

Dyspnea

Difficult or labored breathing; shortness of breath.

Pulmonary embolism

A blood clot in the lung; usually starts when a blood clot travels from a vein in the legs to the pulmonary artery, causing sudden shortness of breath.

blood thinners for a blood clot. If it is determined that your shortness of breath is caused by stress or anxiety, an antianxiety medicine such as lorazepam may be prescribed. Other medicines that are sometimes used are corticosteroids and the pain medicine morphine. Morphine helps people breathe better by slowing the breathing rate and thereby allowing people to take deeper, more effective breaths. If the doctor prescribes medicine for your shortness of breath, do not stop taking it without approval.

Other nondrug measures can help people with shortness of breath. If you have low oxygen in your blood, your doctor will prescribe oxygen (see Question 47). Some breathing exercises, such as diaphragmatic breathing, altering breathing rhythm, and pursed lip breathing, can help people decrease shortness of breath. These breathing exercises also help you to take slower, more effective breaths. Ask your nurse to provide you with instructions for breathing exercises.

If you have shortness of breath, you may be more comfortable sitting up and using pillows for support. Reclining chairs are helpful for sleeping and allow you to be in a semisitting position. Schedule rest periods at regular intervals during activities to relieve shortness of breath. Sometimes an open window or a fan in the room is helpful.

Call your doctor or nurse if you have any of the following:
- Sudden difficulty breathing or inability to catch your breath
- Worsening shortness of breath despite your treatments
- Discomfort or pain in the chest when breathing

- **Bloody or discolored phlegm (sputum)**
- **Difficulty sleeping when lying down**
- **Fever of 100.5°F or more**

Mary Ann's comment:

I get a little panicked when my breathing gets difficult. I am lucky that it only happens on humid days or days with high pollen counts. I never had asthma or any breathing issues until my lung cancer manifested. What helps me is my twice-a-day inhaler (Advair) and an emergency inhaler (Proventil), which I try not to use unless I really, really need it. I have also gained a great deal of weight, which is not helping my breathing as I am lugging 100 pounds extra around every time I move. My appetite is low; so I suspect that the medications I am on may be helping me hold onto this excess weight (along with no exercise). However, I'd rather take my medication and be here to complain about those days I am uncomfortable! Air conditioning has been my source of relief during the pollen-filled humid days.

47. How do I know if I need oxygen?

Oxygen is essential for cells to function normally in the body. Not all shortness of breath is caused by low oxygen. To test for low oxygen, a small device called a *pulse oximeter* is placed on your finger. If it shows that you have a low oxygen level, your doctor will prescribe oxygen and determine how much of it (referred to as liters of oxygen) you need.

Oxygen can be provided for you at home by a respiratory or home care company. Your health insurance provider may cover the cost of it.

Oxygen comes in different types of containers. There are cylinders that contain oxygen. Alternatively, a small machine that pulls oxygen from the room air can be set up at home and plugged into an electrical outlet. The oxygen travels through a tube that extends from the unit and that is attached to another tube (called a *nasal cannula*), placed in your nostrils. Also available are small portable units that are relatively easy to use outside the house.

Take great care when oxygen is in the home. Oxygen itself is nonflammable, but materials will burn more readily in the presence of increased oxygen. When oxygen is not in use, the container should be turned off. Under no circumstances should matches, lighters, cigarettes, or candles be used in the room where oxygen is used or stored. Additionally, oxygen containers should not be stored near gas or electrical heating elements. Your respiratory therapist or the company that provides the oxygen will review other safety measures with you and with your family or caregivers.

Take great care when oxygen is in the home.

48. What should I do if I cough up blood?

If you cough up blood, call your doctor or nurse. Coughing up blood or blood-tinged sputum from the lower respiratory tract (below the throat) or lungs is called **hemoptysis**. Sometimes the phlegm (sputum) is tinged or streaked with blood, and at other times people cough up bright red blood. If possible, estimate the amount of blood that has been coughed up (e.g., one tablespoon, one-half cup), and note the color (e.g., bright red, dark, like coffee grounds).

If you cough up blood, call your doctor or nurse.

Hemoptysis

Coughing up blood or blood-tinged sputum from the lower respiratory tract (below the throat) or lungs.

There are many causes of hemoptysis—a blood clot in the lung, tuberculosis, heart problems, and pneumonia—but the most common is infection, such as bronchitis. In some instances, cancer can also cause hemoptysis.

Sometimes it is difficult to tell if the blood is coming from the lungs, the back of the mouth, or the stomach (vomiting of blood, or hematemesis). Describing other symptoms that you have and the color of the blood can help the physician make a diagnosis.

The doctor may also:

Coagulation profile
A blood test that analyzes the clotting ability of the blood.

- Order certain tests such as a complete blood count (CBC) (analysis of the blood components) or **coagulation profile** (analyzes the clotting ability of the blood).
- Want a specimen of your sputum to determine whether infection is present.
- Order a chest x-ray or CT (commonly referred to as a "CAT" scan) to check for abnormalities in the lungs.
- Look at your lungs and air passages directly through a scope (bronchoscopy).

Treatment of hemoptysis depends on its cause and on the amount of blood coughed up. When hemoptysis is mild and infection is suspected, antibiotics are usually prescribed, along with a cough suppressant (codeine) because coughing can cause irritation and aggravate hemoptysis. For most patients, the conservative measures usually stop the problem.

NUTRITIONAL PROBLEMS

49. I never feel hungry and am concerned about losing weight. What can I do to increase my appetite and maintain my weight?

Weight loss, a common problem for people with cancer, can occur for many reasons. Having cancer changes your metabolism; so you need more calories each day than you usually consume. You may find that you have a poor appetite or that you feel full after eating only a few bites of food. Food may taste differently, and symptoms such as nausea, gas, constipation, pain, fatigue, or emotional distress can further decrease your appetite. Changes in your mouth from the disease or from the treatment may make it difficult to chew and swallow adequate amounts of nutrients and fluids. Finally, changes in how you digest or absorb food may make it difficult for your body to use the nutrients and fluids you are able to take in.

Try very hard to take in adequate amounts of food and fluids to provide energy to your body and to help you tolerate your treatment. Try to maintain your usual weight or minimize the amount of weight you lose. Even if you are overweight when you begin treatment, it is generally not recommended to diet at this time. You can do a number of things to improve your appetite and help maintain your weight.

Medication may be helpful if you have symptoms that are affecting your appetite, like mouth sores, nausea, vomiting, diarrhea, constipation, pain, or emotional distress. If you have any of these problems, ask your doctor for appropriate medication.

Make changes in your diet to maximize the amount of nutrients you take in each day. Here are some suggestions:

- Eat small amounts of food and fluids at a time. Eat six or eight snacks throughout the day rather than trying to eat three full meals. Always have food nearby to nibble on.
- Select foods high in protein and calories. Foods that many people find easy to eat when they are not very hungry are:

Select foods high in protein and calories.

97

- ○ Eggs
- ○ Cottage cheese or yogurt
- ○ Peanut butter
- ○ Sandwiches with sliced turkey or tuna fish
- ○ Baked or broiled chicken, fish, or beef
- ○ Soups
- Add a variety of things to recipes to add calories, such as butter, honey, jelly, sour cream, cheese, yogurt, cream, and evaporated milk. *Eating Hints for Cancer Patients: Before, During, and After Treatment*, published by the National Cancer Institute, provides many helpful recipes (www.cancernet.gov/cancertopics/eatinghints).
- Limit the amount of fluids you take with your meals so that you don't fill up on the fluid.
- Have a limited amount of beverages with caffeine (e.g., coffee, tea, many sodas) because these dehydrate you.
- Have a limited amount of carbonated beverages because these make you feel full.
- Replace fluids with no nutritional benefit, like soda, with fluids that provide nutrients, like cream soups, shakes, and fruit smoothies.
- Try nutritional supplements that are available in your local drugstore: canned drinks, powders to be mixed with water or milk, or puddings. Experiment with different brands to find products you enjoy. Your doctor or nurse may recommend specific supplements for you. You can also use Carnation® Instant Breakfast®, blending it with milk and adding ice cream, yogurt, and/or fruit.

Other suggestions that may be helpful are as follows:

- Ask your doctor or nurse if it is safe for you to have a glass of wine or beer or a cocktail before your meal. Many people find that alcohol stimulates their appetite.

- Avoid eating alone. Having company can make eating more enjoyable, and we often eat more when eating with someone else.
- See Question 50 for suggestions to improve your intake of food and fluid if you are having problems related to changes in taste and Question 52 for suggestions if you are having problems related to swallowing.

If you still have trouble with your appetite despite these measures, ask your doctor if an appetite stimulant would be safe for you to take. Megace® ES, a medicine approved for people with severe weight loss from AIDS, is also used for people with cancer who have lost a lot of weight and are having trouble gaining it back.

Family members and friends often have suggestions and want to give you advice. They may recommend special diets, high-protein drinks, or supplemental megavitamins and antioxidants. Do not take these without first speaking with your doctor or nurse because they may interfere with your treatment or may be dangerous for you.

Family members, who work hard to prepare special foods only to have you push it away after only a few bites, can become frustrated. To avoid conflicts, remind them that you are able to eat only what your appetite allows. Eating should be pleasurable; eat what you want when you want it. You may find it helpful to speak with a *nutritionist*, that is, a registered dietitian who is certified by the American Dietetic Association. Ask your doctor or nurse for a referral to a nutritionist with expertise in working with people who have cancer.

> **Call your doctor if, for any reason, you are unable to eat or drink for more than a day.**

50. Nothing tastes the way it used to, and sometimes I have an awful taste in my mouth. What can I do for this?

Pete's comment:

I have been on chemotherapy for over a year. For several days following treatment, most food tastes very bland and unappetizing. I also have the sensation of feeling slightly queasy. For this period, I have changed my diet to include spicy foods, drink plenty of ginger ale, switch from coffee to tea, and eat smaller, more frequent meals. This approach has enabled me to maintain my weight and actually get more variety into my diet. I also take Prilosec twice a day to help digestion.

Changes in how food tastes and smells can be caused by certain medicines (e.g., antibiotics), some types of chemotherapy, radiation therapy to the head and neck, and surgery in the mouth or head and neck area. The cancer itself can also cause changes in taste. Changes for any reason can be a problem if, as a result, you decrease your food intake and lose weight. If you are getting treatment for your cancer, you have to maintain your weight based on good nutrition.

Most people have four taste sensations: salty, sweet, bitter, and sour. These sensations may be exaggerated by the treatment for your cancer, making foods taste differently than they normally would. In addition, some people note a persistent metallic or bitter taste, and some people note a lack of taste. These changes can be worse if you have a dry mouth (see Question 53 for tips on handling a dry mouth) or a change in your sense of smell. Chemotherapy medicines that most often cause alterations in taste are cisplatin, cyclophos-phamide, doxorubicin, fluorouracil, paclitaxel, and vin-cristine. For most people, these changes in taste are temporary and go away when the treatment is fin-ished, but they may persist for weeks to months.

You can try several things to improve the flavor of your food. One of the most important is to maintain good oral hygiene. This measure includes brushing your teeth on a regular basis and using a mouthwash four to five times a day. Rinsing your mouth immediately before eating, to moisten the taste buds on your tongue, is particularly helpful. Solutions people use include plain water, table salt and water, baking soda and water, or commercial mouthwashes like Biotène. Do not use a mouthwash that contains alcohol because it causes dryness and may worsen the problem. Your doctor or nurse can recommend a mouth care regimen. You can also ask your dentist for recommendations.

One of the most important things you can do is maintain good oral hygiene.

You can do several other things to enhance your appetite and food flavor.

- Always eat foods that look and smell good to you.
- If you have an aversion to the smell of food in gen-eral, ask a family member to cook or grill outdoors for you.
- Use a fan in the kitchen to eliminate or reduce cooking odors.
- Eat foods that are cold or at room temperature to reduce the smell.
- If food has a metallic taste, use plastic utensils to prepare and eat food.
- Try marinating or basting meat or poultry with fruit juices or wine to improve their taste.
- If food is bland, add herbs or other seasonings to enhance the flavor.

For more suggestions, the National Cancer Institute has a booklet entitled *Eating Hints for Cancer Patients: Before, During, and After Treatment* (www.cancernet. gov/cancertopics/eatinghints). This booklet addresses changes in sense of taste and smell, as well as the management of other eating problems. You can also order the booklet over the phone by calling the Cancer Information Service. Your doctor or nurse can suggest other eating hints or refer you to a registered dietitian.

Some studies have shown that taking zinc can improve the taste of food in people who've had radiotherapy to the head and neck area. Zinc may also be beneficial in people getting other treatments for cancer. Before taking any medication to improve the flavor of food or enhance your appetite, including zinc, check with your doctor or nurse.

51. What can I do for mouth sores?

Pete's comment:

Right from the start, I was worried about mouth sores. I switched to Biotène mouthwash, which I use in the morning and evening. I also continue to brush my teeth three or four times a day and drink plenty of fluids. Fortunately, I have been free of mouth sores since starting treatment.

Chemotherapy or radiation therapy destroys tumor cells by preventing them from dividing. Normal cells that divide rapidly are also sensitive to these treatments. With certain chemotherapy drugs and with radiation therapy to the head and neck region, the mucous membranes lining the inside of your mouth and throat may be affected. They may become reddened and feel tender, sore, or painful. You may even develop **oral mucositis**, which is an inflammation or irritation of the mucous membranes in the mouth; this

Oral mucositis

Inflammation or irritation of the mucous membranes in the mouth; can be caused by chemotherapy or radiation therapy.

can be caused by chemotherapy or radiation therapy. Some chemotherapy drugs are much more likely than others to cause mouth sores. If you develop severe mouth sores, your doctor may reduce the chemotherapy dose for your next treatment.

Keep your mouth clean and moist to prevent infection. Brush your teeth with a soft-bristled toothbrush for at least 90 seconds at least two times per day, rinse regularly with a bland rinse to remove loose debris, and keep your mouth moist. Bland rinses can be:

Keep your mouth clean and moist to prevent infection.

- *Saltwater solution:* You can buy normal saline at a drugstore or make this at home, mixing 1/2 teaspoon of salt in a glass of warm water.
- *Sodium bicarbonate solution:* Mix 1/2 teaspoon of baking soda in a glass of warm water.
- *Combination salt and soda solution.*
- *Biotène® Mouthwash*, which you can buy at a drugstore.

Do not use any commercial mouthwash that contains alcohol because it can irritate your mouth. When you use the rinses, swish these in your mouth for at least 10 seconds and then spit.

If you wear dentures that are not fitting correctly, you are more likely to get mouth sores from the rubbing and irritation of the dentures. This may be a problem, particularly if you have lost weight recently; your gums may have shrunk, changing the fit of your dentures. If you are unsure about the fit of your dentures, see your dentist to adjust them if needed.

If you have mouth or throat sores, the membranes may become infected. This is most commonly caused by *Candida*, a type of fungus. Your mouth may look very red, and you may see white, cheesy-looking patches on the membranes or tongue. If you notice these, ask your doctor or nurse to examine you and, if you have *Candida*, a fungal infection, to prescribe an antifungal medication.

See Question 52 for suggestions on managing pain from mouth sores and on ensuring that you eat and drink enough even if you have pain with swallowing.

> **Call your doctor if you are unable to eat or drink for more than a day because of painful mouth sores or if you develop white, cheesy-looking patches in your mouth.**

52. What can I do for difficulty or pain with swallowing?

Swallowing food and liquid may be difficult or painful for a variety of reasons. Surgery or a tumor in the mouth, throat, or esophagus may alter the muscles and other tissues or may cause a blockage in the pathways for swallowing. If you are getting chemotherapy or radiation therapy to the head and neck region or to the chest, you can develop irritation or sores on the mucous membranes lining the inside of your mouth, throat, or esophagus (see Question 51). Certain medications like steroids may increase your risk of developing an infection in your mouth, particularly with *Candida*, a type of fungus, which may cause pain when you swallow.

If you are having pain or difficulty when you swallow, changes in what you eat and drink may be helpful:

- Eat soft or pureed foods that are easy to chew and swallow.

- If you are having difficulty swallowing solid foods, drink the liquid nutritional supplements that are available in your local drugstore. Experiment with different brands to find products you enjoy. Your doctor or nurse may recommend specific supplements for you.
- If you are having difficulty swallowing fluids, try thick cream soups, shakes, fruit smoothies, Jell-o®, ice cream, and frozen juices to be sure you get enough liquid during the day.
- Avoid hot foods or liquids.
- Avoid foods and liquids that can irritate the membranes, such as alcohol, citrus, tomatoes, spices, and rough coarse foods.
- Avoid smoking.

Swallowing will cause pain if your mouth or throat becomes sore or painful. Let your doctor or nurse know so that something can be prescribed for you. A variety of medications may be used, including topical anesthetic medications you can swish in your mouth to numb the membranes (e.g., lidocaine), products that coat the membranes to protect them (e.g., GelClair), and combination mouthwashes (sometimes called "magic mouthwash"). Palifermin (keratinocyte growth factor) is a new medicine used for severe mucositis, a common complication in patients who have had a bone marrow transplant. If your mouth is very painful, a narcotic medication may be needed. If your lips become irritated, vitamin A and D ointment can be soothing.

If you are having difficulty swallowing your medications, ask your doctor to prescribe a liquid version if it is available. If not, many medications can be crushed and mixed with a small amount of juice or applesauce to make them easier to swallow. Check with your pharmacist before crushing any medication because this may affect how the medication works.

If you are unable to swallow enough food and fluid to maintain your weight, your doctor may recommend that you get a **feeding tube**, which is a tube placed through the nose or through the abdominal wall into the stomach to give liquid nutritional supplements. The supplements are instilled through the tube every few hours throughout the day. You can get all the nutrients and fluids you need through this tube.

Some people develop difficulty swallowing after radiation therapy to the head and neck because of changes in the tissues in the back of the throat. Speech therapists can teach you techniques to improve your swallowing. If you develop swallowing difficulties after treatment, ask your doctor or nurse to refer you to a speech pathologist.

> Call your doctor if you are unable to eat or drink for more than a day because of pain or difficulty swallowing.

53. What can I do for my dry mouth?

Dry mouth (*xerostomia*) occurs when the glands that make saliva don't work effectively. This condition can result from radiation therapy or surgery to the head and neck area, from some chemotherapy drugs, from certain medications (e.g., many of the medications used to treat high blood pressure and depression, antihistamines, and decongestants), and from medical problems like diabetes, Parkinson's disease, Sjögren's disease, and HIV or AIDS. If you don't have enough saliva (spit) to

Feeding tube

A tube placed through the abdominal wall into the stomach to give liquid nutritional supplements.

keep your mouth moist, your mouth and throat may feel uncomfortably dry, your sense of taste may change, it may be difficult to chew and swallow food, and speech may even be difficult. A loss of saliva can also cause increased dental decay and an increased chance of developing infections in your mouth.

You can do a number of things to manage a dry mouth:

- Keep your mouth moist. Take frequent small sips of liquids throughout the day and suck on ice cubes of frozen water or juice.
- Use a saliva substitute, like Biotène Oral Balance Moisturizing Gel.
- Avoid tobacco, alcohol, and caffeine, all of which can dry the mouth.
- Take sips of fluids while eating, and moisten foods with gravy, sauce, broth, or yogurt to make them easier to swallow.
- Try to stimulate the glands to produce more saliva by chewing sugar-free gum or sucking on sugar-free hard candies.
- Ask your doctor about medications that can stimulate more saliva. If your glands are able to produce saliva but are not working properly, medication such as pilocarpine may help.

Avoid tobacco, alcohol, and caffeine, all of which can dry the mouth.

To prevent dental decay, brush your teeth after each meal using fluoride toothpaste. You should see a dentist regularly because of your increased risk for dental decay. Your dentist may recommend a fluoride gel to use at night.

For additional information, the National Oral Health Information Clearinghouse of the National Institutes of Health provides a free publication, *Dry Mouth*, which you can find on the Internet (www.nidcr.nih. gov/OralHealth/Topics/DryMouth) or obtain by calling 866-232-4528. Additional information can be found at www.chemocare.com.

DIGESTIVE PROBLEMS

54. What can I do to help with heartburn?

Heartburn is a sensation of burning in the chest, most commonly felt behind the breastbone. Some people describe a sensation that food or liquid is coming back up into the throat, and some describe an acid or bitter taste in the back of their throat, "acid indigestion." Heartburn has nothing to do with the heart and is actually caused by a backflow, or *reflux*, of the digestive stomach acids into the esophagus, where they irritate the lining of the esophagus.

The most common cause of heartburn is GERD, or gastroesophageal reflux disease. This condition develops when the muscle at the lower end of the esophagus does not work properly. This muscle is in the form of a ring, or sphincter. It opens to allow food to pass from the esophagus into the stomach; at other times, it tightens and stays closed to prevent stomach contents from flowing backward into the esophagus. If the muscle does not close properly, there is reflux, resulting in symptoms of so-called "heartburn."

Heartburn may also be caused by increased pressure on the stomach. The pressure may be from excess weight or from a tumor or fluid in the abdomen or pelvis pushing up against the stomach. Other causes include certain medications, foods, and fluids that increase the acidity of the stomach, as well as hiatal hernia (a weakening of the diaphragm muscle, causing part of the stomach to rise into the chest).

> You can take a number of steps to treat heartburn; however, if you have heartburn lasting more than 2 weeks or occurring more than two times a week, call your doctor. If untreated, reflux can cause serious problems, such as ulceration in the esophagus, scarring and narrowing of the esophagus, and even changes in the cells of the membranes lining the esophagus that put them at risk of developing into a cancer.

Changes in your diet are helpful. Avoid foods that are known to bring on heartburn: citrus, tomatoes, onions, garlic, fatty foods, mint, and pepper. Avoid caffeinated, alcoholic, carbonated, and citrus beverages that may also bring on heartburn. Eat small portions of food at a time, and do not eat at bedtime.

Positioning also plays a role. Sit upright when eating and drinking, and do not lie down or bend over at the waist for at least 2 hours after eating a meal. Elevate the head of the bed 6 to 8 inches if you have symptoms when lying down. Avoid wearing clothes that are tight around the belly, and, if you wear a belt, keep it loose.

A variety of medications are helpful in treating heartburn. Some are available over the counter and some require a prescription.

- *Antacids* are salts of aluminum, magnesium, calcium, or a combination of these, which neutralize acid. They work quickly but last only up to 2 hours.
- *Histamine receptor antagonists* (*H₂ blockers*) reduce the production of acid by blocking histamine, one of the

chemicals that stimulates the stomach to make acid. These generally take about 30 to 60 minutes to work and may last up to 10 hours. H_2 blockers include cimetidine, ranitidine, famotidine, and nizatidine.

- *Proton pump inhibitors (PPIs)* reduce the production of acid by blocking the pump that makes the acid. PPIs include omeprazole, lansoprazole, and esomeprazole. These generally take about 60 minutes to work but may last up to 24 hours.

H_2 blockers and PPIs may be used regularly to prevent problems. Before taking any medication, ask your doctor or nurse which medication is best for you, how much to take, and how often to take it. The Heartburn Alliance has additional information on this problem (www.heartburnalliance.org).

55. What can I do to manage nausea and vomiting?

Lisa's comment:

I was lucky not to experience the classic "nausea or vomiting" side effect associated with chemotherapy. However, my gastrointestinal side effects manifested with a "heavy gut" feeling—I felt like I swallowed a bunch of rocks. It would start the day after treatment and last about 3 days. By my fourth cycle of therapy, the feeling would start the night before (anticipatory). Eating helped my symptoms somewhat. I was on so many antinausea drugs, I could not help think that my symptoms were related to them. All and all, I figured it was better to have the "heavy gut" rather than the actual nausea and/or vomiting. I could tolerate these symptoms because I knew once I got off the adriamycin/ cyclophosphamide, the paclitaxel would be easier to tolerate.

Nausea and vomiting have long been considered unavoidable side effects of cancer treatment. However, with the development in recent years of new antinausea medications (antiemetics), this is no longer the case.

Radiation therapy to the abdominal area and a variety of chemotherapy drugs may cause nausea or vomiting. Either can result from irritation of the stomach or from chemical stimulation of areas in the brain that trigger nausea and vomiting. *Nausea* is often experienced as feeling sick to your stomach or feeling queasy. *Vomiting* is when you throw up stomach contents through your mouth. Retching, gagging, or dry heaves feel similar to vomiting, but no stomach contents come up.

People vary widely in their reactions to the same treatment. Some people have very distressing nausea or vomiting, some have mild symptoms, and some have none at all. For people who experience nausea or vomiting, the timing of the symptoms also varies. Some people develop symptoms within minutes or hours after treatment, and some develop symptoms days later. For some people the symptoms last several hours, and for others they persist for many days. For some people, the most severe symptoms occur before leaving home in the morning or while on the way to treatment; this is called *anticipatory* nausea or vomiting.

Of the many effective ways to manage nausea and vomiting, the most important is the use of medication. See Question 56 for a review of the medications available.

There are also ways to manage nausea or vomiting that do not rely on medication. Using body and mind techniques can be very helpful, particularly with anticipatory nausea or vomiting. Examples of these techniques are guided imagery, self-hypnosis, and progressive muscle relaxation. If you are interested in learning one of these techniques, ask your doctor or nurse for a referral to someone trained in the related field. Another helpful strategy is to minimize the use of things in the home with particularly strong odors, like perfumes or certain cleaning products.

Changes in what you eat and drink may also help in managing nausea and vomiting. Here are some specific suggestions:

• Eat a light meal before each treatment.
• Eat small amounts of food and liquids at a time.
• Eat bland foods and liquids.
• Eat dry crackers when feeling nauseated.
• Limit the amount of liquids you take with your meals.
• Maintain adequate liquids between meals; take mostly clear liquids such as water, apple juice, herbal tea, or bouillon. Some people find that carbonated sodas are helpful; others do better drinking soda without the fizz.
• Eat cool foods or foods at room temperature.
• Avoid foods with strong odors.
• Avoid high-fat, greasy, and fried foods.
• Avoid spicy foods, alcohol, and caffeine.

Taking in adequate amounts of fluids and nutrients is important for your health. If you feel that seeing a nutritionist would help you select appropriate foods, ask your doctor or nurse for a referral. For additional information on managing nausea and vomiting, the National Comprehensive Cancer Network has guidelines for patients at www.nccn.org.

> **Call your doctor or nurse if you are unable to keep any food or fluids down for 12 hours or if you are taking in only minimal amounts for 24 hours.**

56. What medications are available to treat nausea and vomiting?

A number of medications are available to treat nausea and vomiting, and several new ones have recently been developed. Given the new ways of using and combining these medications, nausea and vomiting can be prevented or well controlled in most people. Medications used to prevent or treat nausea and vomiting are called **antiemetics**.

These medications are most commonly given orally, intravenously, or by rectal suppository. Depending on the specific treatment you are getting and on the timing and severity of your symptoms, your doctor will prescribe a specific antinausea medication for you. You may be instructed to take the medication at home before coming for treatment, the nurse may give you medication immediately before your chemotherapy, or you may be instructed to take the medication on a schedule at home after your treatment. Sometimes, depending on the type of your treatment, the doctor will give you a combination of two or three medicines. For example, if you are getting chemotherapy that is likely to cause moderate to severe nausea or vomiting, your doctor may prescribe one or two medications for the nurse to give you before your treatment and medications for you to take at home afterward. The various antinausea medications work in different ways; so if one medication is not effective, call your doctor or nurse and ask for something else.

Antiemetics
Medication used to prevent or treat nausea and vomiting.

Here are some of the medications most commonly used to treat nausea and vomiting related to cancer or cancer treatment:

Medication	How Taken
For Moderate to Severe Nausea and Vomiting	
Granisetron (Kytril)	Tablet or IV
Ondansetron (Zofran)	Tablet or IV

113

Aprepitant (Emend)	Tablet
Dolasetron (Anzemet)	Tablet or IV
Dexamethasone (Decadron)	Tablet or IV
For Mild Nausea	
Prochlorperazine (Compazine)	Tablet, injection, or suppository
Metoclopramide (Reglan)	Tablet or injection

In addition, lorazepam (Ativan) can be given either intravenously or by mouth if you experience anticipatory nausea.

Many of these medications can cause constipation. See Question 58 on tips to manage constipation.

Nausea and vomiting can be effectively treated; let your doctor or nurse know if you are having persistent symptoms. For more information on nausea and vomiting, visit the National Cancer Institute's website (www.cancer.gov/cancertopics/pdq/supportive-care/nausea/Patient/page4).

57. What can I do to manage diarrhea?

Chemotherapy and radiation therapy destroy tumor cells by preventing them from dividing. Normal cells that divide rapidly are also very sensitive to these treatments. Certain chemotherapy drugs and radiation to the abdominal or pelvic area will cause the mucous membranes lining the small intestine to become thinner and lose their ability to function as effectively as normal. As a result, the intestines do not absorb fluid and nutrients adequately and do not easily digest lactose (the sugar in milk). In addition, the muscle layer of the intestine may become overactive, moving the intestinal contents through the bowel more quickly than usual. All this may result in abdominal cramping and diarrhea. Some chemotherapy drugs are much more likely than others to cause diarrhea.

There are many effective ways to manage cramping and diarrhea. Antidiarrheal medications such as loperamide (over-the-counter Imodium A-D) or Lomotil (prescription) are very effective. Your doctor or nurse will instruct you on how to take these medications.

Changes in what you eat and drink will also help in managing diarrhea. Some specific suggestions follow:

- Eat small amounts of food and liquids at a time.
- Eat bland foods and liquids.
- Increase the amount of fluid you drink when having diarrhea.
- Drink a variety of liquids, selecting clear liquids you can see through, like apple juice, cranberry juice, herbal teas, and Jell-o.
- Sports drinks with electrolytes are particularly good to take, as well as fat-free broth or bouillon.
- Eat bananas, applesauce, canned cooked fruits with skin removed, white potatoes without the skin, cooked squash or carrots, and tomato paste or puree (without chunks of tomato). Bananas and white potatoes are good sources of potassium, which is important to replace when having diarrhea.
- Avoid liquids with alcohol and caffeine.
- Avoid high-fiber foods.
- Avoid whole-grain breads and cereals. Instead have white bread, pasta, noodles, cold cereals of corn or rice, saltines, and white rice.

- Avoid raw fruits (except bananas) and vegetables, cooked vegetables that cause gas, and beans.
- Avoid foods high in lactose, such as milk, ice cream, and soft cheeses. Instead, have lactose-free milk, hard cheeses, yogurt, and sorbet.
- Avoid fatty, greasy, fried foods, like cream sauces and gravies. Limit the amount of butter and oil you use.

Taking in adequate amounts of fluids and nutrients is important for your health. If you feel that seeing a nutritionist would help you in selecting appropriate foods, ask your doctor or nurse for a referral.

> **Call your doctor or nurse if your diarrhea does not respond within 12 hours to the medications you are taking and to changes in your diet. If you have severe diarrhea and are not able to replace the fluid you lose, you can become severely dehydrated.**

Mary Ann's comment:

Diarrhea is one of the side effects of the chemo I am on. Don't be ashamed to share this information with your doctor or nurse practitioner. There are wonderful, prescription medications that really help control this uncomfortable problem.

58. What can I do to manage constipation?

Lisa's comment:

Constipation was probably my biggest complaint with treatment—related to my antinausea medications. Although intellectually I was prepared, my actual discomfort was incomprehensible. I drank fluids, I took stool softeners and laxatives, but I still had difficulty. I never had to succumb to the big guns (lactulose) but probably would have if my therapy with adriamycin/cyclophosphamide continued.

About 95% of patients with cancer have constipation at some point during the course of their treatment. This condition may present as infrequent bowel movements, incomplete emptying of the bowels, the passage of hard stool, or discomfort or difficulty in passing stool.

Cancer can cause constipation in a number of ways. If a tumor grows in or around the colon or rectum, it may block the passage of stool. If a tumor compresses the spinal cord, it may damage the nerves that stimulate the emptying of the bowel. If a tumor causes changes in blood chemistry, the stool may slow down as it passes through the intestine. Cancer treatments can also cause constipation. Certain chemotherapy drugs (e.g., vinblastine, vincristine, vinorelbine), antinausea medications, and pain medications can slow the movement of stool through the intestine. Patients with cancer may have to reckon with many other causes of constipation: increasing age, decreased physical activity, inadequate fiber in your diet, inadequate fluid intake, not taking the time to move your bowels, a variety of medications, and certain medical conditions like diabetes, hypothyroidism, Parkinson's disease, and depression.

If you feel you are constipated, describe your symptoms to your doctor or nurse. Tell them how often you pass your stools, the consistency of the stool, if it is painful when you have a bowel movement, and whether you have any abdominal pain or cramping.

You can do a variety of things to prevent and treat constipation.

- Form regular daily routines to help train your bowel. Try to move your bowels at the same time each day.

Form some regular daily routines to help train your bowel.

117

Many people feel the strongest urge right after breakfast. When you feel the urge to move your bowels, go right away; try not to hold it in.

- Daily exercise, especially walking, helps stimulate stool movement within the intestines.
- Changes in your diet can also help with constipation. Drink six to eight glasses of fluid a day. Add fiber to your diet, and include fruit, vegetables, whole grains, and high-fiber cereals.

When changes in daily routine and diet are not enough, a variety of medications are available to help with constipation. Many of these can be purchased over the counter, but some require a prescription. Taking a combination of a stool softener (e.g., docusate) and a laxative (e.g., senna, bisacodyl, lactulose, polyethylene glycol) on a regular basis can help. Ask your doctor or nurse which medications you should take, what dose, and how often you should take these.

URINARY PROBLEMS

59. What can I do for frequent urination?

Frequent urination is the need to urinate (void) more often than every 2 hours or more than eight times in a 24-hour period. Frequent urination that occurs at night is called **nocturia**. Some people feel as though they have to void again just after they have finished going to the bathroom. Frequent urination may be accompanied by other symptoms. Urgency is the sudden, sometimes uncontrollable need to urinate; this may be so strong that people leak urine before they reach the bathroom. Some people also have pain, burning, and/or a change in the color of the urine (cloudy or bloody).

Nocturia

Frequent urination that occurs at night.

There are several causes of frequent urination:

- Increase in fluid intake
- Diuretics (water pills, such as furosemide)
- Diabetes
- Urinary tract infection (UTI)
- Urinary retention (when the bladder does not fully empty all urine)
- Benign prostatic hypertrophy (BPH), an enlargement of the prostate gland that makes it difficult for the bladder to empty
- **Cystitis**, an inflammation or irritation of the bladder that can be caused by radiation therapy to the pelvic area, chemotherapy instilled into the bladder to treat bladder cancer, or certain chemotherapy drugs given through a vein (cyclophosphamide or ifosfamide)

Cystitis
Inflammation or irritation of the bladder.

Frequent urination can interfere with your normal daily routine, causing you to stay home more than you normally would, and it can interrupt sleep, making you more tired than usual. If you have frequent urination, discuss the condition with your doctor or nurse. Tell them when it started, how many times you urinate during the day and night, and if you have any other symptoms in addition to the frequency. They may ask for a sample of urine to test for infection. Other tests (e.g., CT scan, ultrasound) may be performed depending on the symptoms you have and on the results of the urine tests.

Diuretic
A medication that increases the production of urine; also called a "water pill."

Drink 1 to 2 quarts of fluids every day.

Most cancer patients are encouraged to drink 2 to 3 quarts of fluid per day. This by itself will cause frequent urination. To avoid waking in the night to urinate, stop drinking fluids about 3 to 4 hours before you go to sleep. If you are taking a **diuretic** (a medication that increases the production of urine, also called a "water pill"), check with your doctor to see if you can take it earlier in the day to reduce the need to urinate at night.

If you have diabetes and your sugar is very high, you will urinate more often. Make sure that you take your medications and check your sugar according to your doctor's instructions.

Infection is one of the most common causes of frequent urination in people with cancer. Urinary tract infections (UTIs) are usually associated with other symptoms, such as burning or pain on urination, pain in the back (flank pain), cloudy or foul-smelling urine, or urine that is dark yellow or has blood in it. Sometimes people also have lower abdominal pain and a fever. If the urinalysis and urine culture show that you have an infection, the doctor will prescribe an antibiotic.

> **If you have symptoms of a urinary tract infection, a fever above 100.5°F, and/or shaking chills, call your doctor immediately.**

If an enlarged prostate gland (BPH) is causing frequent urination or if you have urinary retention from some other cause, your doctor may prescribe medicine for you or refer you to a **urologist** (a specialist in problems or diseases of the urinary tract).

Urologist
A specialist in problems or diseases of the urinary tract.

If your urinary frequency is from radiation therapy and/or chemotherapy, the symptoms should get better with time after the treatment is completed. Your doctor may prescribe medication to help in the meantime. For example, oxybutynin may be prescribed to reduce bladder spasms.

Continue to drink enough fluid during the day. Decreasing or eliminating alcohol and caffeine will also help. Keep up with your usual activities, and do not stay at home all the time. Try to urinate on a set schedule. Keep a diary of when you urinate during the day and when you drink fluids to help you plan activities outside the house. Plan bathroom breaks.

For more information on urinary problems and BPH, contact the American Urological Association Foundation (www.urologyhealth.org).

60. What can I do for burning with urination?

Pain or burning on urination, usually caused by irritation or infection of the bladder or urinary tract, is called **dysuria**. It may be accompanied by other symptoms, such as frequency, urgency, and nocturia (see Question 59 for more information). A vaginal infection or a rash in the area can cause burning when you urinate from skin irritation. The causes of dysuria are:

- Urinary tract infection (UTI)
- **Prostatitis**, an inflammation or infection of the **prostate gland** in men (The prostate gland is a gland within the male reproductive system that is located just below the bladder surrounding part of the urethra, the canal that empties the bladder, and that produces a fluid that forms part of semen.)
- Cystitis, an inflammation or irritation of the bladder that can be caused by radiation therapy to the pelvic area, by chemotherapy instilled into the bladder to treat bladder cancer, or by some chemotherapy drugs given through a vein (cyclophosphamide or ifosfamide)

Dysuria

Pain or burning on urination, usually caused by irritation or infection of the bladder or urinary tract.

Prostatitis

Inflammation or infection of the prostate gland in men.

Prostate gland

A gland within the male reproductive system that is located just below the bladder surrounding part of the urethra, the canal that empties the bladder, and that produces a fluid that forms part of semen.

121

If it is determined that you have a urinary tract infection (see Question 59) or prostatitis, your doctor will prescribe antibiotics. You should also drink at least 2 quarts of fluid each day.

Cyclophosphamide and ifosfamide can cause irritation of the bladder, resulting in burning and sometimes blood-tinged urine. To prevent this condition, you will be given extra intravenous fluids with the chemotherapy and instructed to drink large amounts of fluid for 1 to 2 days afterward. You will also be asked to empty your bladder on a regular schedule. If you are getting ifosfamide, your doctor will also prescribe an intravenous medicine, called Mesna, that protects the lining of the bladder.

Radiation therapy to the pelvis can also cause irritation to the bladder with burning, frequency, and urgency. This can begin 3 to 5 weeks after the start of treatment and usually subsides 2 or more weeks after completion. Irritation of the bladder from chemotherapy or radiation therapy is managed in a similar way. Increase the fluid that you drink to 1 to 2 quarts every day and

Avoid alcohol and caffeine.

avoid alcohol and caffeine. If you have pain on urination, your doctor may prescribe a medicine called phenazopyridine (Pyridium). This medicine is a local analgesic that specifically works on the lining of the bladder to reduce the burning or pain. It will make your urine dark yellow or orange, and it can stain your clothing.

> **If you have burning with urination with a fever above 100.5°F, shaking chills, flank pain, severe abdominal pain, or frank (visible) red blood or blood clots when you urinate, call your doctor.**

61. *What can I do for incontinence?*

Incontinence is the uncontrolled loss or leakage of urine. Anything that interferes with the muscles of the bladder or pelvic floor or the nerves in this area can affect your ability to control urine flow. There are different types of incontinence.

Incontinence
The uncontrolled loss or leakage of urine.

- *Stress incontinence* occurs when you leak urine when you sneeze, cough, laugh, or exercise. This is usually from weakened pelvic floor muscles.
- *Urge incontinence* results when you lose urine because you cannot get to the bathroom in time.
- *Overflow incontinence* occurs when the amount of urine exceeds the bladder capacity, causing leakage.
- Or you may just have no control over urination and lose large amounts of urine all the time.

Incontinence, if bad enough, can keep you from enjoying your normal activities and can cause skin irritation and breakdown. Here are some of the causes of incontinence:

- Aging and childbirth, which can cause weakening of the pelvic floor muscles
- Urinary tract infection or inflammation
- Surgery to remove the prostate for an enlarged prostate gland (BPH) or prostate cancer
- Neurologic problems, such as metastasis (spread) of cancer to the spinal cord

If you have incontinence, describe the symptoms as clearly as you can to the doctor. The physician may order certain tests and in some cases recommend that you see a urologist, a doctor who specializes in urinary problems.

> **If you are incontinent of urine and have back pain or difficulty walking or moving your bowels, call your doctor.**

Problems with Breathing, Nutrition, Digestion, and Urination

Depending on the cause, incontinence may be a short-lived or permanent problem. Incontinence from infection or inflammation usually goes away when the condition resolves. Incontinence from prostate surgery, neurologic problems, childbirth, or aging can last several months or in some cases be permanent.

You can do several things to help with incontinence. The first is to keep a diary of when you have loss of urine. If you notice that this occurs every 2 hours, then try to urinate every hour and a half, whether you feel the need to urinate or not. If this is successful, you may be able to train your bladder and increase the length of time between visits to the bathroom. It is also important to continue to drink the amount of fluids prescribed by your doctor. To avoid incontinence at night, stop drinking fluids 4 to 5 hours before bedtime.

Kegel exercises

Exercises that are designed to increase muscle strength and elasticity in the pelvis and that may be recommended for treatment of urinary incontinence.

Ask your doctor or nurse to teach you **Kegel exercises**, which are exercises that are designed to increase muscle strength and elasticity in the pelvis and that may be recommended for treatment of urinary incontinence. These are performed by squeezing (contracting) the same muscle that you use to stop urinating. If you perform this exercise regularly, you may be able to improve your control over urine flow.

Keep your skin clean and dry. Regularly wash your genitals, groin, buttocks, and upper thigh skin with soap and water to remove any urine. Your doctor or nurse can prescribe lotion to protect the skin in this area. Additionally, pads or briefs with absorbent material can help protect your skin. Change them as soon as they become wet. If you notice redness, rash, or breakdown of skin in this area, notify your doctor or nurse.

If your incontinence is caused by an overactive bladder muscle (detrusor muscle), your doctor may prescribe medication such as propantheline, oxybutynin, and tolterodine. These relax your bladder muscle and allow it to hold more urine, decreasing the urge to urinate. You have to take this medicine exactly as prescribed.

Depending on the cause, your doctor may recommend that you see a urologist (a specialist in urinary problems). The urologist may recommend a surgical procedure or teach you how to catheterize yourself. Catheterization involves inserting a thin tube through the urethra into the bladder and allowing the urine to drain. For more information on incontinence, contact the National Association for Continence (www.nafc. org or 800-252-3337).

PART SIX

Appearance and Sexual Issues

I have gained weight from my cancer treatment.
What can I do to lose it?

I don't feel the desire to be sexually intimate
with my partner the way I used to.
What can I do to maintain our relationship?

Will I be able to conceive a child after treatment?

More . . .

62. I have gained weight from my cancer treatment. What can I do to lose it?

Most people believe that a diagnosis of or treatment for cancer will cause them to lose weight. However, many people actually gain weight. The gain can be from the cancer, the treatment for cancer, or side effects of cancer treatment.

Some cancers cause you to accumulate large amounts of fluid. **Fluid retention** is a condition in which the body does not eliminate adequate fluid and can cause swelling and weight gain. Accumulation of fluid in the abdomen is called *ascites* (see Question 77). This can be seen in advanced cancers of the ovary, colon, or liver and in metastatic cancer to the liver. Accumulation of fluid in the tissues with swelling is called **lymphedema** (see Question 76). This is most commonly seen in an arm or leg, after removal or damage to lymph nodes, from surgery or radiation therapy.

Some chemotherapy treatments, for example, high-dose cisplatin, require you to drink a lot of fluid or to be given large amounts of intravenous fluids. You may notice that you gain weight after these treatments. Usually, your body will eliminate this fluid on its own, several days after chemotherapy.

Docetaxel is a type of chemotherapy that, when given in repeated doses, can commonly cause you to retain fluid. Your doctor will prescribe dexamethasone (a steroid) before and after docetaxel to prevent fluid retention. You have to take this medicine as directed.

Steroids are medications that are used to relieve inflammation and, in people with cancer, to prevent allergic reactions from chemotherapy and to ease other

Fluid retention

A condition in which the body does not eliminate adequate fluid and can cause swelling and weight gain.

Lymphedema

A condition in which lymph fluid collects in tissues, usually in an arm or leg, after the removal or damage to lymph nodes, from surgery or radiation therapy.

Steroids

Medications that are used to relieve inflammation and, in people with cancer, to prevent allergic reactions from chemotherapy and to ease other problems, such as nausea and vomiting, pain, shortness of breath, trouble breathing, and loss of energy.

problems, such as nausea and vomiting, pain, shortness of breath, trouble breathing, and loss of energy. Steroids can increase your appetite and cause you to retain fluid. Thus, long-term treatment with steroids (taken every day) can also bring on weight gain.

Some treatments for cancer can cause mild nausea or indigestion (heartburn). Frequent snacks often relieve these symptoms but may result in weight gain. There are medicines to help reduce nausea and indigestion, reducing the need to eat increased amounts of food. See Questions 54 to 56 for more information on the treatment of heartburn and nausea.

Excessive weight gain can make it difficult to get around, cause added stress on your legs and joints, and make you short of breath. Additionally, weight gain can affect the way you feel about your appearance. If you gain weight while you are getting treated for cancer, tell your doctor or nurse. If your weight gain is from fluid retention, your doctor may prescribe a diuretic (a water pill), which helps your body eliminate the excess fluid.

If your weight gain is caused by overeating, simple measures such as eliminating second helpings, eating smaller portions, and eliminating sweets and fried foods may help you lose weight. While you are getting treatment for cancer, you need to eat a well-balanced diet even if you want to lose weight. Fad diets and herbal weight-loss products are not recommended because they may be unhealthy. Your doctor or nurse can refer you to a dietitian or nutritionist to help you with diet and weight loss.

Exercise is also important to help lose weight or prevent weight gain and has other benefits for people who are getting cancer treatment as well (see Question 34). Exercise does not need to be strenuous or complicated. Even taking a daily walk is good for you and will help you to lose or maintain your weight.

63. My body seems different now that I have cancer. I don't feel as attractive as I used to. What can I do to feel better about myself?

Lisa's comment:

I was never big on makeup. One of the first things my fellow nurses got excited about post-mastectomy was, "Oh, now you get to go to Look Good, Feel Better." I did attend the class, learned some cosmetic tips, and got my free bag of goodies. I pretty much didn't do anything else with the stuff.

The prospect of losing my hair was upsetting. I knew all along that I didn't want to wear a wig. I figured I would wear a baseball cap, scarf, or bandana. My hair loss occurred during the hot summer months, so the bandana was perfect. The actual hair loss was disgusting. I had cut my hair semishort so I wouldn't have to clean up long hair. I couldn't believe how much hair kept falling off my head!

I must say I never felt unattractive. I just felt I stuck out like a sore thumb. That was something I didn't expect. I suppose if I wore a wig I probably wouldn't have felt that way.

Many people feel aware of changes in their body when they have been treated for cancer. Some things can be seen, like scars from surgery, drainage tubes, venous catheters, loss of hair, or a change in weight. However, other things are not visible at all, just a feeling that your body is different and knowing that things inside are not the way they used to be. In addition, you may not be able to do all of the things you used to do at work or at home or for enjoyment. These changes may all affect how attractive you feel as a man or woman.

Although there may be no way to reverse these physical changes, you can take measures to feel better about how you look. Selecting clothes that make you feel good can make a big difference. You may want to have favorite clothes altered to fit better if you have gained or lost weight. Some women find that using makeup, having a manicure or pedicure, or wearing scarves helps them feel better about how they look. The Personal Care Products Council, the National Cosmetology Association, and the American Cancer Society sponsor a free program, "Look Good, Feel Better," that is dedicated to helping men and women being treated for cancer feel better about their appearance. They teach techniques that help restore your appearance and enhance your self-image. They provide many tips on their Internet site and present group programs all over the country. To find out if it is available in your area, check their Internet site (www.lookgoodfeelbetter.org) or call 800-395-LOOK.

Also, think about what makes you who you are as a person. Is it the way you look? Is it what you do? Is it what you have accomplished in the past? Is it your relationships with other people? Is it those intangible things in your mind, your heart, and your soul? While recognizing that some things have changed since your diagnosis with cancer, recognize those things that still make you who you are. Think about the accomplishments of your life. Plan time to be with people you enjoy. Continue to involve yourself in the things that give you intellectual satisfaction. Maintain a connection with your source of spirituality. All these actions help to remind you of who you are as a person and enhance your feelings about yourself.

Appearance and Sexual Issues

64. I don't feel the desire to be sexually intimate with my partner the way I used to. What can I do to maintain our relationship?

Physical intimacy is one aspect of a loving relationship. It gives us personal pleasure and creates a feeling of closeness with our partner. Sexual intercourse is one way of being physically intimate. However, you may find that pain, fatigue, emotional distress, or the side effects of treatment affect your desire for sex or your ability to enjoy sex.

If you would like to continue having sexual intercourse with your partner, consider strategies that will make it more pleasurable for you. Take medications that have been prescribed for any symptoms that are bothersome to you. Select a time of day when you usually have more energy and when you know you will have privacy. Experiment with different positions that might be more comfortable or less tiring. Of course, be sure always to use a safe method of birth control if there is a risk of pregnancy.

You can maintain a physically intimate relationship with your partner in many ways without having intercourse. Cuddling, hugging, touching, rubbing, and holding hands are some of the ways you can feel close. Talk with your partner about your relationship, your fears and concerns, and your hopes and desires. This can create a feeling of intimacy between you and help you experience pleasure being together.

Talk with your partner about your relationship.

Discuss your concerns with and ask questions of your doctor and nurse. They can explain how your disease and treatment may affect your sexuality. Sex therapists can counsel you. You can get a referral from your doctor or nurse or from the American Association of Sexuality Educators, Counselors and Therapists (www. aasect/org). In addition, the American Cancer Society has two excellent books that can be helpful: *Sexuality for the Woman with Cancer* and *Sexuality for the Man with Cancer.*

65. I have developed menopause from my treatment. How can I manage the symptoms?

Menopause is the cessation of menses (menstrual period) for a period of 12 consecutive months and results from the loss of ovarian function. The ovaries normally produce hormones called estrogen and progesterone, and, when the ovaries stop making these hormones, menstruation stops. The average age for beginning menopause is 51.

Radiotherapy to the pelvis and some types of chemotherapy can damage the ovaries. As a result, some patients stop menstruating during treatment. For many, menstruation will begin again a number of months after treatment has ended. However, some women will develop premature or early menopause as a result of their treatment. Symptoms may occur very soon after starting treatment or months or years later. The surgical removal of both ovaries induces permanent menopause and immediate symptoms.

Symptoms of menopause vary from person to person; they can be more intense in younger women with medically-induced menopause. The most common symptoms are:

- Hot flashes (or flushes) and/or night sweats
- Sleep disturbances or insomnia
- Mood swings, depression, and anxiety

- Decreased memory and concentration
- Dryness, itching, and burning of the vagina and labia
- Decrease in sexual desire

Osteoporosis

A condition characterized by a decrease in bone mass and density (thinning of the bones), causing bones to become fragile.

Additionally, after menopause, women are at increased risk of coronary heart disease and of **osteoporosis** (a condition characterized by a decrease in bone mass and density [thinning of the bones], causing bones to become fragile).

Not all women will have symptoms from menopause, and if you do have symptoms, most of these will go away over time without any treatment. Hormone therapy may be indicated for some women to manage severe symptoms from menopause. This treatment may involve using estrogen alone (for women who have no uterus) or a combination of estrogen and progesterone (with progesterone protecting the uterus). Risks come with taking hormone therapy, and it is not recommended for women with some types of cancer, unexplained vaginal bleeding, or a history of blood clots, liver disease, or cardiovascular disease. Whether to take hormone therapy is a decision that you and your doctor will make together.

Some women take certain complementary therapies for symptoms of menopause, like herbs, "natural" products, or dietary supplements (e.g., soy products and black cohosh). At this time there is not enough information to recommend herbs or natural products for menopausal symptoms. Studies are currently being performed to determine the benefits and risks of these products. See Question 18 to learn how to get information about specific complementary therapies. Talk to your doctor or nurse before taking any medicine or herbal product (over-the-counter or prescription) for menopausal symptoms.

Other measures may help you cope with menopausal symptoms.

- For suggestions on how to manage hot flashes, see Question 66.
- For difficulty sleeping, establish a regular sleep schedule, going to bed at the same time each night. Avoid heavy meals in the evening and keep the bedroom dark, cool, and quiet.
- For mood swings, depression, or anxiety, try to identify the sources of stress in your life and address them if at all possible. Take time for yourself, and plan activities with family and friends with whom you enjoy spending time. Regular exercise, such as walking or gentle aerobics, and relaxation techniques may be helpful. Talk with your doctor about antianxiety or antidepressant medication to help for persistent symptoms.
- For vaginal dryness or discomfort during sexual intercourse, vaginal moisturizers, such as Replens, and vaginal lubricants, such as Astroglide or K-Y Jelly, may be helpful (see Question 67). Your doctor or nurse can tell you how to use these products. Ask your doctor about the use of a vaginal estrogen cream or vaginal estrogen tablets. See Question 64 if you are concerned about the loss of sexual desire.
- Your doctor or nurse can also make recommendations for the management or prevention of osteoporosis and for the prevention of coronary artery disease.

Here are some resources for additional information about menopause and management of menopausal symptoms:

- *North American Menopause Society:* www.menopause. org or 440-442-7550
- *The National Women's Health Information Center:* www.4women.gov
- *National Institutes of Health*: www.nhlbi.nih.gov/ health/women/index.htm

66. How can I manage hot flashes?

Lisa's comment:

I was diagnosed with breast cancer at 40 years of age—premenopausal. After two cycles of adriamycin/ cyclophosphamide chemotherapy, over the course of one month, I experienced three unusual menstrual periods. Then the hot flashes started and my menses ended. The hot flashes intensified once I started tamoxifen therapy (postchemotherapy). I would awaken four to five times in the night, completely soaking wet. I have been on tamoxifen for 3 months now, and night sweats no longer awaken me. I have hot flashes throughout the day, but they are tolerable.

Hot flashes (or flushes) are the most common symptom in women around the time menopause begins, whether from natural aging or induced prematurely from cancer treatment (see Question 65). They are thought to be caused by a decline in estrogen and other hormones. Hot flashes can also occur in men, as part of the normal aging process if there is a decline in the male hormone testosterone.

Hormonal therapies used for breast and prostate cancers that stop the body from producing male or female hormones or that block the activity of these hormones (see Question 9) can also cause hot flashes. Usually, the frequency of the hot flashes decreases over time.

During a hot flash, you may feel warm or hot, and you may perspire or have "sweats." Your skin will feel warm and may become red. Hot flashes can occur any time during the day, but they occur most often at night, and may affect your sleep. Hot flashes typically last for more than 1 year and in some people they can last for as long as 5 years. For some people they are very uncomfortable.

Identify and avoid those things that trigger hot flashes, such as alcoholic beverages, hot drinks, and spicy foods. For some women, slow deep breathing at the onset of a hot flash helps. Dress in layers, so that, if you feel a hot flash starting, you can remove a layer of clothing and later add it back, as needed. Cotton clothing may be more comfortable against the skin because it more readily absorbs perspiration than synthetic clothing.

Some women report that a variety of over-the-counter herbal and dietary products are helpful, but we have no scientific evidence that they are effective. However, a number of prescription medicines have been found to be helpful. These all have side effects; so you need to discuss the options with your doctor before making a decision about trying them. Studies have shown that antidepressants such as fluoxetine (Prozac), venlafaxine (Effexor), and paroxetine (Paxil) are effective in reducing hot flashes in both men and women. Usually, the doses used to treat hot flashes are lower than those used to treat depression; so the chance of side effects is lessened. Gabapentin (Neurontin) is an antiseizure medicine that has also reduced the frequency and severity of hot flashes in both men and women.

Hormone therapy may be an option for some women, especially those with very severe hot flashes and other distressing menopausal symptoms. For more information, see Question 65.

Appearance and Sexual Issues

Information regarding management of hot flashes can be found at:

- *The National Women's Health Information Center:* www.4women.gov
- *National Institutes of Health:* www.nhlbi.nih.gov/ health/women/index.htm

Treatment recommendations for men with hot flashes are limited, but some information can be obtained at:

- *American Cancer Society:* www.cancer.org
- *Prostate Cancer Foundation:* www.prostatecancerfound ation.org

67. My doctor said there would be changes in my vagina after treatment. What does this mean, and how can I treat this?

Vaginal changes can occur when a woman produces less estrogen. Estrogen keeps the vagina moist and gives it the ability to elongate and become wider during sexual activity. A decrease or loss of estrogen causes vaginal dryness, thinning of the vaginal walls, and irritation. As a result, you may be more prone to vaginal yeast infections and urinary tract infections (see Question 59), and you may have vaginal bleeding from irritation during intercourse. In addition, the vaginal walls lose their ability to stretch, causing vaginal tightness. After pelvic radiation or some types of gynecologic surgery, you may develop scar tissue in the area and experience vaginal shortening and narrowing. These changes may cause pain or discomfort during sexual intercourse (called **dyspareunia**) and may make it difficult for you to have a thorough pelvic examination.

Before you start treatment for your cancer, speak to your doctor or nurse about the vaginal changes that

Dyspareunia

Pain or discomfort during sexual intercourse.

can occur as a result of your treatment. Ask for ways you can minimize or prevent some of these changes.

Vaginal dryness or irritation can be helped by using vaginal moisturizers such as Replens or Senselle, which can be used every night or every other night. You should use a moisturizer even if you are not having sexual intercourse. When having intercourse, you may also want to use a vaginal lubricant to avoid discomfort. It is best to use a water-based, fragrance- and color-free product such as K-Y Jelly or Astroglide. Avoid oil-based products, such as mineral oil or Vaseline. Some women have even found that use of a spermicidal jelly or natural yogurt relieves discomfort during intercourse. Warming the lubricants or moisturizers in warm water before use can make them comfortable to use. Vaginal dryness or irritation can also be helped by wearing loose-fitting cotton panties and pants. Avoid douching because these may cause further vaginal dryness and irritation.

Hormone therapy or vaginal creams or rings with estrogen may also provide relief from vaginal symptoms. Hormonal medicines require a prescription, and they are not used in women with certain types of cancer. You should discuss the advantages and disadvantages of using these products with your doctor or nurse. See Question 65 for more information on hormone therapy.

Vaginal discharge, burning, and itching may be signs of a vaginal infection. Some types of vaginal infections can be passed on to your sexual partner during sexual activity. If you develop these symptoms, contact your doctor or nurse, who will prescribe a medication, usually a vaginal cream, to eliminate the infection. Sometimes your partner may also need to be treated with medication.

If you have had certain types of gynecologic surgery or pelvic radiation, you should stretch the vaginal walls on a regular basis to prevent narrowing and shortening. Using a dilator three times a week can accomplish this. Vaginal dilators are easy to use. Your doctor or nurse will tell you how to get a dilator and give you instructions on how to use it and when to begin after radiotherapy or surgery.

For more information, the American Cancer Society has an excellent booklet called *Sexuality for the Woman with Cancer.*

68. Will I be able to conceive a child after treatment?

Lisa's comment:

I never felt that I wanted to have children. This decision and reality were acceptable because I wasn't married. At forty and single, being diagnosed with breast cancer and having to undergo chemotherapy and then tamoxifen therapy, I was faced with the permanence of my prebreast cancer reality. I would never have children. I was surprised by my sudden concern and inner turmoil about being childless. Having the choice taken away from me was very upsetting, and I still get emotional thinking about it.

For many people, the ability to have a child is one of the most important aspects of their lives, and the loss of fertility after cancer treatment can be a significant source of distress. The ability to conceive a child is a complicated process that depends on the production of healthy sperm and eggs, as well as on functional reproductive structures that enable a woman to carry a fetus to term and deliver a healthy baby. Reproductive problems can affect both men and women and can be

Reproductive problems can affect both men and women.

140

caused by cancer or cancer treatment. In addition, with increasing age, women are more likely to have difficulty conceiving.

If you have cancer and want to have children in the future, speak to your doctor or nurse before you begin treatment. If you are at risk of infertility from treatment, options are available for many men and women to preserve their fertility and be able to conceive a child after treatment is completed.

For men, sperm banking is an option and, if desired, should be done before any cancer treatment begins. Ask your doctor or nurse to give you the name of a sperm bank in your area. Sperm banking usually involves collecting three separate specimens of semen over a week to 10 days, but, with new technologies for assisting with reproduction, only one specimen may be adequate. You shouldn't have to delay your treatment. This procedure requires a semen sample, which is usually obtained by masturbation. The ejaculated semen is collected in a special container. The sperm are then analyzed, frozen, and stored. After treatment, if you want to start a family, the sperm are thawed and used to fertilize your partner's eggs. Health insurance usually does not cover sperm banking, and the costs vary from one sperm bank to another; call a few banks to help you decide where to go.

For some women, freezing of embryos is an option. Women take hormone injections for about 2 weeks to stimulate the ovaries to produce an increased number of mature eggs. These are then removed from the ovaries and fertilized in the laboratory (in vitro fertilization, IVF) with her partner's sperm (or sperm from a donor). The cells from the resulting embryos begin

Options are available for many men and women to conceive a child after treatment for cancer.

Appearance and Sexual Issues

141

to divide and multiply, and after 3 to 5 days the healthy embryos are frozen and stored. When a woman wants to try to have a child, the embryo is thawed and transferred into her uterus. For women who have no partner at the time they are going to begin cancer treatment and do not want to use donor sperm, egg freezing may be an option. These are fertilized later, when the woman wants to use them to become pregnant. For women who are not able to carry a child, the embryo can be transferred into the uterus of a gestational carrier or surrogate.

For women not able to collect eggs before treatment and not able to conceive after treatment, IVF can also be used with donor eggs from another woman. The eggs can be fertilized by your partner's sperm, producing embryos, and transferred into your uterus or into the uterus of a gestational carrier or surrogate.

IVF requires a delay in treatment of about 2 to 6 weeks. Before beginning this process, speak with your doctor to be sure the delay will not be dangerous for you. IVF is expensive, and many insurance companies don't cover it. Nevertheless, ongoing advancements in these assisted reproductive technologies are enabling more and more women to be able to have children after cancer treatment.

The decision that you and your partner make regarding having a family is a very personal one. Remember that there is no one right decision. Some people may decide to use the available reproductive technologies, some may decide not to have children, and still others may decide to adopt. Facing treatment for cancer is difficult, and concerns about the ability to have a family can add to the stress.

When learning more about fertility related to cancer and cancer treatment and finding sperm banks and reproductive centers in your area, the following resources are helpful:

- *Fertile Hope:* www.fertilehope.org (This organization also provides financial assistance for those who meet specific criteria.)
- *My OncoFertility:* www.myoncofertility.org
- *Lance Armstrong Foundation:* www.livestrong.org
- *American Society for Reproductive Medicine:* www.asrm.org

69. I'm not able to get or maintain an erection since my treatment. How can this be treated?

The inability to get and/or maintain an erection is called *erectile dysfunction* (*ED*). Cancer and treatment for cancer (radiation therapy and surgery) may affect erectile function. Multiple studies have shown that sexual functioning is an important aspect of quality of life for men with cancer. Sexuality and physical intimacy are ways that men and women express themselves in intimate relationships, and erectile dysfunction may inhibit intimacy.

The sexual response in men involves four phases. First is the desire for intimacy. Second is excitement. Nerves stimulate blood vessels in the penis to dilate or open up; the increased blood flow in the penis causes it to become erect, or "hard." The third phase is orgasm, a "climax" or "coming." This is the sensation of pleasure and the time when semen is pushed out of the penis, causing an ejaculation. The fourth and final phase is when blood drains out of the penis, causing it to lose its erection.

Appearance and Sexual Issues

There are many causes of erectile dysfunction in men with cancer, and ED can occur as part of the normal aging process. The causes of erectile dysfunction include:

- Surgery for cancer in the pelvis
- Radiation therapy to the pelvis
- Hormonal therapy for cancer
- Symptoms from cancer or cancer treatment
- Changes in your body that alter how you feel about yourself

With some types of cancer surgery in the pelvis, the nerves involved in getting and maintaining an erection are removed or injured. With new **nerve-sparing techniques** the nerves are left undisturbed with the goal of maintaining erectile function. Before having surgery for prostate, colorectal, or other cancers of the genital or urinary tract, speak to your surgeon about the chances of nerve injury and if it is possible to have nerve-sparing surgery.

Radiation therapy to the pelvis may injure the nerves and blood vessels that cause blood to flow into the penis, resulting in erectile dysfunction. Hormonal therapy for prostate cancer reduces the testosterone level, resulting in a loss of desire for sex and erectile dysfunction. In addition, symptoms from cancer or cancer treatment, such as fatigue, nausea, and pain, and changes in how you feel about yourself, can cause a loss of desire for sex, resulting in an inability to have an erection.

If you are having problems getting or maintaining an erection, speak to your doctor or nurse, who may want to do a blood test to check your hormone levels. The

Nerve-sparing surgeries

Surgical procedures for men with prostate cancer in which the prostate is surgically removed and the nerves are left undisturbed with the goal of maintaining erectile function.

treatment recommended depends on the results of a physical examination, blood testing, and your prior medical and sexual history. Treatments include prescription medicine (Viagra, Levitra, Cialis), vacuum constriction devices, penile injections, and permanent penile implants. Professional counseling or sex therapy may also be helpful. Your doctor or a specialist in erectile dysfunction (urologist) can help you determine your best option.

For more information, the American Cancer Society has an excellent booklet on Sexuality for the Man with Cancer.

Appearance and Sexual Issues

PART SEVEN

Neurologic Problems, Fluid Retention, and Blood Chemistry

What is cerebral edema? How is this managed?

Why are my legs swollen? What can I do to minimize the swelling?

I have heard that some people can get diabetes from their treatment. How is this diagnosed and treated?

More . . .

NEUROLOGIC PROBLEMS AND INFLAMMATION

70. What is peripheral neuropathy and how is this managed?

Lisa's comment:

My experience with peripheral neuropathy was surprising. As an oncology nurse (16 years) I have taught the signs and symptoms of chemotherapy toxicities thousands of times. So you would think I'd recognize a symptom. With my first paclitaxel treatment I noticed that my hands and wrists were itchy about 3 days after therapy. I would be at work and I'd go crazy scratching. I was out to lunch with a coworker one afternoon and started complaining about my weird itching sensations localized to the wrists/hands, and she said, "You're having peripheral neuropathies." I was shocked. Over the years, I'd never heard one patient complain of pruritis in the "glove" area only. By my last paclitaxel cycle, the classic numbness and tingling presented itself in both my hands and feet. However, the symptoms improved a few weeks off treatment.

Peripheral neuropathy

A condition of the nervous system that causes numbness, tingling, burning, or weakness; usually begins in the hands or feet and can be caused by certain anticancer drugs.

Peripheral neuropathy is a condition of the nervous system that causes numbness, tingling, burning, or weakness; it usually begins in the hands or feet and can be caused by certain anticancer drugs.

The *peripheral nerves* are the nerves outside the brain and spinal cord. When there is damage to the peripheral nerves, the symptoms depend on which type of peripheral nerves is affected.

There are three types of peripheral nerves:

* *Sensory nerves* allow us to feel temperature, pain, vibration, and touch.

- *Motor nerves* are responsible for voluntary movement; they allow us to walk and open doors, for example.
- *Autonomic nerves* control involuntary or automatic functions, such as breathing, digestion, sweating, and bowel and bladder function.

Peripheral neuropathy can occur in people with diabetes, alcoholics, and patients with severe malnutrition. Some antibiotics (e.g., ciprofloxacin, levofloxacin) can cause peripheral neuropathy. In people with cancer, the most common cause of peripheral neuropathy is chemotherapy. Chemotherapy can affect any of the peripheral nerves but the most common are the sensory nerves, causing numbness and tingling in the hands and feet. The following chemotherapy medicines can cause damage to peripheral nerves: paclitaxel, docetaxel, cisplatin, oxaliplatin, vincristine, vinorelbine, and thalidomide. If you have peripheral neuropathy from another cause, chemotherapy can sometimes make it worse.

In people with cancer, the most common cause of peripheral neuropathy is chemotherapy.

The symptoms of peripheral neuropathy are:

- Numbness and tingling ("pins and needles") in the hands and/or feet
- Burning pain in the hands and feet
- Difficulty writing or buttoning a shirt
- Difficulty holding a cup or glass
- Constipation
- Decreased sensation of hot and cold
- Muscle weakness
- Decreased hearing or ringing in the ears (tinnitus)

Oxaliplatin causes a unique symptom from peripheral neuropathy in almost half of all patients who take the drug. It is an acute sensitivity to cold that starts anywhere from hours to 1 to 2 days after treatment and can last up to 14 days. If you are on oxaliplatin, do not suck on ice chips or drink cold fluids, and use a straw when drinking. Do not take anything from the freezer or touch cold metal objects unless you have gloves on. Cover your mouth, nose, and head with a scarf when going outdoors in cold weather.

Preventing chemotherapy-induced neuropathy is difficult, but if you get it, it is possible to prevent it from getting worse. If you have any of the symptoms before you start chemotherapy or if you develop them while on chemotherapy, tell your doctor or nurse. Describe the symptom, tell them when it started, and whether the symptom makes it harder or prevents you from performing any activities, like writing a check, buttoning your shirt, or walking. Because chemotherapy can sometimes cause permanent neuropathy, be sure to talk about this before your treatment.

Often the diagnosis of peripheral neuropathy is based on a description of your symptoms and on a physical examination. Blood tests cannot diagnose peripheral neuropathy, and usually other tests are not needed. Sometimes your doctor may ask you to see a **neurologist**, who is a physician who takes care of people with problems or diseases of the nervous system.

Neurologist

A physician who takes care of people with problems or diseases of the nervous system.

If you have neuropathy and it is interfering with your activity or causing pain, your doctor may decide to reduce the dose of chemotherapy or stop it altogether. With the therapy stopped, the neuropathy should not get worse and may even go away. Neuropathy can take from 6 to 12 months to get better or to resolve completely.

Your doctor may also prescribe medication. The medicines most commonly prescribed are also used to treat seizures and depression: gabapentin (Neurontin), carbamazepine (Tegretol), pregabalin (Lyrica), and amitriptyline (Elavil). Amitriptyline makes people sleepy, and it should be taken at bedtime. If pain is associated with your neuropathy, your doctor may prescribe an opioid (see Question 25 on pain medicine).

If you have peripheral neuropathy, you can take advantage of several safety hints so you don't hurt yourself.

- If you have numbness and tingling in your feet and have trouble walking or if you trip often, keep your home well lighted, avoid scatter rugs, and watch the placement of your feet when you walk.
- Use handrails when walking on stairs.
- If you drive a car, make sure you can feel the pedals with your feet.
- If you have trouble feeling temperature, ask someone else to test the temperature of drinks or bathwater so that you don't burn yourself.

Your doctor or nurse may refer you to a physical or occupational therapist to help you to regain function.

For more information on peripheral neuropathy in people with cancer, refer to The Neuropathy Association at neuropathy.org and to Oncolink at oncolink.org (search "neuropathy").

71. What is cerebral edema? How is this managed?

Cerebral edema is a swelling of the brain from inflammation or other diseases. Of the many different causes of cerebral edema, two are stroke and head injury.

Cerebral edema

Swelling of the brain from inflammation or other diseases.

In patients with cancer, the most common causes are primary brain tumors (tumors that start in the brain) or metastatic brain tumors (tumors that start elsewhere and spread to the brain). Carcinomatous meningitis can also cause cerebral edema. This condition is caused by cancer cells that "seed," or start growing, on the lining of the brain. Swelling from radiation therapy or surgery to the brain may also cause cerebral edema.

The brain is part of the central nervous system and is protected by the skull. If the brain swells, pressure (*increased intracranial pressure*) can develop because the skull does not expand. The symptoms from this type of pressure are:

- Headache
- Nausea and vomiting
- Blurred or double vision
- Difficulty walking
- Seizures
- Difficulty speaking or finding the right words
- Weakness of an extremity or one side of the body
- Personality changes or difficulty thinking

MRI is the best test to determine whether you have cerebral edema.

If you have any of these symptoms, contact your doctor or nurse. If you think you have cerebral edema, the physician will review your symptoms, examine you, and may order an MRI of the head. MRI is the best test to determine whether you have cerebral edema. If you are claustrophobic or have difficulty taking an MRI, alert your health care providers, who may be able to prescribe helpful medicine. A CT scan of the head may also be needed to determine whether you have another cause of your symptoms.

If you have cerebral edema, treatment depends on the cause, and the goal of treatment is to maintain or restore neurologic function. In nearly every case, steroid medicines are used to decrease inflammation and edema (see Question 72 for more information on steroids). If you have symptoms, they will often improve or resolve once you start steroids. If you have a seizure as a result of cerebral edema, antiseizure medicines are prescribed. If these medicines are given to you, you have to take them exactly as prescribed. In cases of severe edema, special intravenous fluids and surgery are sometimes used to decrease edema; this procedure requires a stay in the hospital.

If you have a primary brain tumor or a tumor that has metastasized to the brain, surgery, radiotherapy, or both are needed. Chemotherapy that goes directly to the brain (regional chemotherapy) is sometimes used to treat carcinomatous meningitis. The chemotherapy is given into an artery or into the cerebrospinal fluid that surrounds the brain.

72. What are steroids? Why are they used?

Steroids are very potent anti-inflammatory medicines that doctors use for a variety of medical problems. In patients with cerebral edema from cancer, steroids are used to decrease the swelling in the brain and to reduce neurologic symptoms caused by the swelling. Steroids are also helpful in preventing nausea and vomiting from chemotherapy and in treating severe allergic reactions. Steroids are usually given in pill form, although sometimes they are given intravenously (by vein). The steroid that is most often used in these situations is dexamethasone. Other steroids that are sometimes used are hydrocortisone, methylpred-nisolone, and prednisone.

Before you start to take steroids, talk to your doctor or nurse about the potential side effects and how to take the medicine. Side effects are more common if you are taking the medicine for a long time. The side effects are:

- Muscle weakness
- Weight gain
- Difficulty sleeping
- Increased blood sugar
- Indigestion or stomach ulcer
- Osteoporosis
- Personality changes
- Increased risk for infection

You can prevent or minimize some of these side effects. To avoid stomach upset or ulcer, always take your steroid medicine with food. Your doctor may also prescribe an antiulcer pill for you to take (e.g., omeprazole or lansoprazole). If you have difficulty sleeping, ask if you can take the medicine early in the day. If you are at risk for osteoporosis, your doctor will prescribe calcium and/or a medicine like alendronate (Fosamax) or pamidronate, which strengthens the bones. If you are at risk for infection, your doctor may give you a special antibiotic. Also, if you have diabetes, steroid use may increase your blood sugar. So your doctor may want to monitor your blood sugar more closely or recommend changes in your diabetes medicines.

If you have been taking the steroid medicine for 2 or more weeks and your doctor feels you no longer need it, he or she will taper you off the medicine slowly. The total daily dose will be reduced slowly over several days to weeks.

> **You have to take the steroid medicine exactly as your doctor prescribes it, and you must not stop taking it abruptly.**

73. I am having trouble remembering things and feel confused at times. What can I do about this?

People with cancer sometimes experience **cognitive dysfunction**, that is, difficulty remembering names, places, or events or trouble with language skills, concentration, or arithmetic. Scientists studying this problem in patients with cancer have found that some degree of impairment is common. Although most of the time the impairment is subtle, it can still be quite bothersome to patients.

Cognitive dysfunction

Difficulty remembering names, places, or events or trouble with language skills, concentration, or arithmetic.

Lisa's comment:

My friends and I would joke about it—"Oh, it's that chemo brain again!" I would forget things they'd tell me or have difficulty verbalizing myself. It was quite frustrating at times, but a good excuse at other times! I definitely see improvement in my cognitive function now that I am off chemotherapy.

There are many causes of cognitive impairment. It may be a direct effect of a tumor in the brain (e.g., cerebral edema, metastatic brain tumor) or a remote effect of a tumor outside the brain (e.g., paraneoplastic syndrome; see Question 81). Treatments for cancer, including chemotherapy, biologic therapy, and radiation therapy, are responsible for cognitive dysfunction in one-third to one-half of patients reporting symptoms. Abnormal blood chemistry, certain medications, fatigue, anxiety, depression, stress, and pain can also contribute to impairment.

The treatment of cognitive dysfunction begins with finding the cause of the problem. If you experience any of the symptoms, call your doctor or nurse, who will review your symptoms and examine you. Blood tests can determine whether the problem is from abnormal blood chemistry; for example, high calcium levels in the blood can cause cognitive impairment. When the blood level is corrected, the problem will resolve. If your difficulty stems from anxiety, depression, or pain, appropriate medicines may be prescribed. If one of your medications, such as a pain medicine or antibiotic, might be causing the problem, your doctor may change it. If the problem is from fatigue and anemia, erythropoietin may be prescribed to treat the anemia (see Question 38). If your cancer turns out to be the source of the problem, then treatment of the cancer may bring relief. If your treatment for cancer is the cause, your doctor or nurse can prescribe other interventions.

Medication is sometimes used. Donepezil hydrochloride (Aricept), a medicine used in treatment for Alzheimer's disease, is helpful in patients with cognitive impairment. Methylphenidate (Ritalin) and modafinil (Provigil) have also been used with some success. If your symptoms are troublesome to you, speak to your doctor about the possibility of having physical, vocational, or occupational therapy and cognitive rehabilitation. These interventions have been helpful for others and may benefit you by improving your daily level of functioning. In addition, many health care professionals and cancer patients have cited the benefits of daily physical and mental activity in helping with cognitive function. For more information on cognitive dysfunction and helpful interventions, consult the American Cancer Society (www. cancersymptoms. org or www.cancer.org; search "chemo brain").

FLUID, BLOOD CHEMISTRY, AND BLOOD VESSELS

74. Why are my legs swollen? What can I do to minimize the swelling?

People with cancer can develop swelling in their legs for several reasons. First, when you have lost a lot of weight, the amount of protein in the blood decreases, causing fluid to leak out of the blood vessels and accumulate in the tissues. The fluid accumulates in the feet, ankles, and legs because gravity pulls the fluid downward. Second, certain chemotherapy drugs and other medications may cause fluid retention. This excess fluid may leak out of the blood vessels and lead to swelling. Third, a tumor in the abdomen or pelvis can put pressure on the lymph vessels and veins coming up from the legs. These vessels—throughout your body—carry fluid that normally collects in the tissues back into the bloodstream. If the vessels become blocked, they lose their ability to carry this fluid out of the tissues, leading to swelling. Finally, **thrombosis** (the formation or presence of a blood clot inside a blood vessel) may form in the veins of the leg, blocking the flow of blood up from the legs. This usually occurs in only one leg, so the swelling is usually seen in only one leg. Thrombosis in a deep vein that is accompanied by inflammation of the vein, causing redness, heat, and/or pain in the leg is a condition known as *deep vein thrombosis (DVT)*. Cancer patients are particularly at risk for this problem, which must be treated medically as soon as possible to prevent serious complications (see Question 75).

Depending on the cause of swelling, a number of strategies may help reduce the swelling and improve your comfort. Be sure your shoes, socks, and pants are

Thrombosis

The formation or presence of a blood clot inside a blood vessel.

Neurologic Problems, Fluid Retention, and Blood Chemistry

157

not too tight because tightness may constrict the vessels in your leg and increase the swelling. You may need to purchase shoes and socks that are bigger than your usual size. If you do not have a blood clot in your leg, you can also purchase special compression stockings at the drugstore, which may improve the ability of the vessels to return excess fluid from the legs. However, these must fit correctly to avoid constriction and worsening of the problem. If you notice indented rings in the leg skin when you remove your socks or stockings, they are too tight. Walking may also be helpful. Walking causes contractions of your leg muscles, which supports the ability of the vessels to return excess fluid from the legs. Try to walk short distances frequently throughout the day, but avoid standing in place for a long time. Whenever sitting, keep your legs elevated. Position them so that your feet are higher than your knees, which are higher than your hips. This way, gravity will help pull the fluid out of your legs. Water pills (diuretics) may be helpful if the swelling is from fluid retention. However, some people may become dehydrated from diuretics; so they should be taken only if prescribed. If the swelling is from fluid retention, reducing the amount of salt in your food may also help.

75. What is deep vein thrombosis (DVT)? How is it diagnosed and treated?

Patients with cancer are at risk for developing *deep vein thrombosis (DVT)*. A blood clot forms in the vein of a leg (thrombosis), blocking the flow of blood up from the leg and leading to swelling. This condition is accompanied by inflammation of the vein, usually causing redness, heat, and/or pain in the leg. If left untreated, the blood clot builds up over time. Pieces of the blood clot (**emboli**) can then break off, travel through blood vessels, and obstruct or block the flow of blood. These can block a blood vessel to one of your vital organs, like the lung (a condition called *pulmonary embolus*).

> **Call your doctor immediately if you develop sudden swelling in one leg, with or without redness or tenderness of the calf.**

If your doctor suspects that the swelling may be from a blood clot, a **Doppler ultrasound** examination of your leg may be ordered. In this simple procedure, high-energy sound waves (ultrasound) are bounced off internal tissues or organs and make echoes that form a picture of body tissues, called a *sonogram*; it is used to determine whether there is a clot in a blood vessel in an arm or leg.

If the diagnosis is confirmed, treatment with anticoagulants is started immediately to prevent the blood from forming additional clots. Over time, the body will naturally break down the existing clot. Heparin is the drug most commonly used initially. In the past, heparin was usually given by continuous intravenous infusion, requiring hospitalization for a number of days, or by injection under the skin with a small needle several times a day. New low-molecular-weight heparin is typically used now, with its several advantages:

- It can be given safely at home with only one or two injections a day.
- The dose can be determined more accurately than with other forms of heparin.
- There is no need to have frequent blood tests to monitor its effects.

Emboli

Blood clots that travel through blood vessels and that can obstruct or block the flow of blood.

Doppler ultrasound

A procedure in which high-energy sound waves (ultrasound) are bounced off internal tissues or organs and make echoes that form a picture of body tissues, called a *sonogram*; used to determine whether there is a clot in a blood vessel in an arm or leg.

Neurologic Problems, Fluid Retention, and Blood Chemistry

Some patients remain on low-molecular-weight heparin; for others, an oral anticoagulant medication, warfarin, is also begun within a day or two of starting heparin. However, warfarin takes several days to a week to reach the right level in your blood. There is no standard dose of warfarin; your dose is determined by its effect on your blood. To determine the dose for you, two blood tests are used: the prothrombin time (PT) and the international normalized ratio (INR). Your doctor will adjust your dose of warfarin until the INR reaches a therapeutic level (between 2 and 3). At that time, the heparin is usually stopped. You will continue on the warfarin for at least 6 months, and you may have to stay on this medication for the rest of your life. Throughout that time you will have to have periodic blood tests, anywhere from twice a week to once a month, to confirm that your dose is correct. Adjustments in the dose are made as needed to keep the INR between 2 and 3.

You have to take the exact dose of warfarin prescribed each night because small changes in the dose can have very large effects on your blood. If you do not take enough warfarin, you can develop more blood clots. If you take too much, you can develop bleeding. If you notice any signs of bleeding, contact your doctor or nurse immediately.

Certain foods can affect the metabolism of warfarin, causing it to have either a greater or lesser effect at the same dose. Ask your pharmacist to give you a list of foods that interact with warfarin, and try to avoid them while on this medication. In addition, warfarin can interact with a variety of medications. Always make sure to tell any doctor who prescribes medication for you that you are taking this drug.

Occasionally, patients develop new or worsening blood clots despite being treated with an adequate dose of warfarin. In this case, your doctor may put you back on heparin on a long-term basis. An alternative treatment involves the use of an **inferior vena cava (IVC) filter**. The inferior vena cava is a large vein that empties into the heart and carries blood from the legs and feet and from organs in the abdomen and pelvis. The filter is an umbrella-like device that is placed in the inferior vena cava to prevent blood clots in the legs from traveling to the lungs.

76. What is lymphedema? How can I manage this?

Lymph is a fluid composed of water and proteins that brings nutrients to the tissues and then is absorbed into the *lymphatic system*, which is a connection of vessels and lymph nodes that carry the fluid back to the bloodstream. *Lymph nodes* are little bean-shaped structures located throughout the body that filter bacteria and waste products from the lymph. A backup or blockage in this system that prevents lymph from returning to the circulatory system can cause swelling (edema) in an arm or leg.

Lymphedema is an abnormal accumulation of lymph fluid caused either by overproduction of lymph (primary lymphedema) or by an obstruction of the lymph vessels or nodes, causing a backup or accumulation of lymph in the tissues beneath the skin (*secondary lymphedema*). Lymphedema can occur anywhere in the body where lymph nodes or lymph vessels are present, but it usually occurs in an extremity (arm or leg), causing it to become swollen. Secondary lymphedema is common in people with cancer, particularly in people who have had removal of lymph nodes as part of their cancer treatment or who have had injury or scarring of the lymph nodes. Lymphedema can cause discomfort or pain, limitations in the use of the swollen extremity, and changes in the appearance of your body. Preventive measures, early recognition, and treatment are helpful in the management of lymphedema.

Risk factors for developing lymphedema are:

- The surgical removal of lymph nodes or vessels in the underarm or groin areas for the treatment and staging of cancer
- Scar tissue development after surgery or radiation therapy to the underarm or groin
- Obstruction from a tumor
- Cellulitis (infection) in the affected extremity
- Obesity

The incidence of lymphedema is lower in the last decade because of improvements in surgical and radiation therapy techniques. Acute lymphedema may occur after surgery, but it usually resolves once the body compensates (i.e., heals itself). Chronic lymphedema can occur from months to years after treatment for cancer. If you have lymphedema, you may experience heaviness, throbbing pain or soreness, and a feeling of tightness from your wristwatch, ring, shoes, or clothes in the affected arm or leg. In addition, your skin may become shiny and tight or brownish in color, and it may feel firm. The other causes of swelling in an arm or leg include the development of a blood clot in a blood vessel (see Question 75) and infection.

Preventive measures, early recognition, and treatment are helpful in the management of lymphedema.

> **Call your doctor or nurse for any new swelling in your arm or leg. State whether you also have any pain, redness, red streaks, fever (over 100.5°F), chills, or shortness of breath.**

If your arm or leg is swollen, your doctor will perform a physical examination and measure the swollen extremity to compare it with your normal one. Other tests might be ordered, such as ultrasound, CT scan, or MRI, which indicate whether the obstruction is in a blood vessel or lymph vessel.

If you have had surgery to remove lymph nodes as part of your cancer treatment, ask your nurse about ways to prevent lymphedema. Here are some prevention strategies:

- Perform gentle strengthening and stretching exercises to keep the affected limb working normally.
- Avoid lifting or moving heavy objects on the side of surgery.
- Keep the skin clean and moisturized, avoid cuts or cracks in the skin, and avoid insect bites.
- Avoid blood draws, intravenous lines, and blood pressure measurement in the affected arm.
- Report signs of infection to your doctor or nurse (redness, tenderness, swelling, fever).
- Report other changes in your limb, including pain, numbness, or changes in skin color.

If you develop lymphedema, several treatments may be helpful. Unfortunately, no medicines are available to prevent or treat lymphedema. Here are possible treatments:

- Elevation of the affected limb
- Use of a compression garment, such as a sleeve or stocking

- Massage
- Compression bandaging
- A pressure pump

It may also be a good idea to see a *lymphedema specialist*, who is usually a physical therapist with additional training in the management of lymphedema. If you have pain or are distressed as a result of your lymphedema, speak with your doctor about prescribing an antidepressant or pain medicine.

For more information on lymphedema, contact the National Lymphedema Network at 800-541-3259 or on the Internet (www.lymphnet.org). There is a special Internet resource for people with lymphedema from treatment for breast cancer (www.breastcancer.org; search "arm lymphedema").

77. What is ascites? How is this treated?

Peritoneal cavity

The space within the abdomen and pelvis that contains many structures, including the intestines and liver, and that is lined by thin membranes.

Ascites is an abnormal buildup of fluid in the **peritoneal cavity**, which is the space within the abdomen and pelvis that contains many structures, including the intestines and liver, and that is lined by thin membranes. The *peritoneum* is a membrane that lines the abdominal cavity; one layer surrounds the abdominal and pelvic organs, and the other layer lines the wall of the abdominal cavity. Normally, a small amount of fluid in this cavity prevents friction during organ movement. In healthy people, this fluid moves constantly in and out of the peritoneal space. In some people, the cancer causes increases in the amount of fluid moving into the space or obstruction of the circulatory and lymphatic systems, causing fluid to back up and become unable to move out of the space. These problems can cause the accumulation of fluid in the peritoneal cavity, called *malignant ascites*. Cancers that can cause malignant ascites are gynecologic tumors (e.g., ovary, uterus), gastrointestinal tumors (e.g., colon, stomach, liver, breast cancer, mesothelioma, and lymphoma). Diagnosis of ascites is accomplished by physical examination and radiologic tests, including ultrasound, CT, and/or MRI of the abdomen.

Symptoms of ascites can vary, depending on the amount of fluid in the abdomen. Small amounts of fluid may cause vague symptoms, whereas large amounts can cause more discomfort and swelling of the abdomen. If you have ascites, you may feel some of the following symptoms:

- Weight gain, with clothing fitting more tightly across the abdomen
- Abdominal bloating, discomfort, or pain
- Decreased appetite
- Indigestion
- Nausea or vomiting
- Shortness of breath
- Fatigue

If you have ascites and these symptoms, you can make yourself more comfortable. If your abdomen is swollen from too much fluid, wear loose clothing. For a decreased appetite, try to eat six small meals every day, instead of two or three large meals. Eat foods that are high in protein and calories. If you have nausea or vomiting, take antinausea medicines on a regular basis and before meals (see Question 56).

> **Call your doctor or nurse if you have ascites and if you:**
> - **Are short of breath**
> - **Have uncontrolled nausea or vomiting or uncontrolled pain**
> - **Are suddenly unable to fit into your clothes**

Your doctor may recommend the removal of fluid from your abdomen.

Paracentesis

A procedure in which a thin needle or tube is placed through the abdominal wall to drain fluid from the peritoneal cavity.

Shunt

Allows fluid to move from one part of the body to another.

In addition to these comfort measures, your doctor may recommend the removal of fluid from your abdomen, which can be accomplished by inserting a thin tube into the peritoneal space where the fluid is located with the help of an ultrasound machine. Once the tube is in the right place to drain fluid, it is attached to a drainage bag. When the fluid is finished draining, the tube is removed and the fluid discarded. This procedure is called a **paracentesis**.

Usually, after paracentesis your symptoms will improve. Unfortunately, the fluid usually reaccumulates in the days to weeks afterward. Paracentesis can usually be performed as needed to relieve your symptoms. For some patients, special tubes can be left in place for a period of time to allow for the continual drainage of the fluid if needed.

Another way to remove fluid from your abdomen involves the placement of a permanent **shunt**, which is implanted or created, and allows fluid to move from one part of the body to another. When a shunt is employed to control ascites, it is placed in the abdomen to direct the fluid into the bloodstream. Once the fluid is redirected into the bloodstream, your kidneys remove it, and you eliminate it with your urine. Your doctor will recommend this procedure if it is right for you.

Sometimes directing chemotherapy into the peritoneal cavity can also help to control ascites.

78. What is a pleural effusion? How is this treated?

Pleural effusion is an abnormal buildup of fluid in the pleural space. The *pleura* are membranes that line the inside of the chest wall and cover the outside of the lungs. The space between the membranes is called the **pleural space**. Normally, this space contains a small amount of fluid, which provides lubrication for the lungs to expand and contract during breathing. Pleural fluid moves into and out of the pleural space. If fluid builds up in this space, the lungs cannot expand normally when you inhale, causing you to have shortness of breath. Pleural effusions can occur in one or both lungs.

Pleural effusions can be caused by:

- Infection (e.g., pneumonia)
- Congestive heart failure
- Surgery in the chest or abdomen
- Cancer
- Certain chemotherapy drugs

Fluid buildup that is caused by cancer is called a *malignant pleural effusion*. Usually, cancer cells cause the buildup either by lodging in the pleura or by being present in the pleural fluid, causing the pleura to become irritated. When this happens, extra fluid can collect in the pleural space. The cancers that most often cause pleural effusions are lung, breast, adeno-carcinoma of unknown primary, mesothelioma, lymphoma, and leukemia.

Not everyone has symptoms from a pleural effusion. If the fluid collection is small, you may not have any symptoms. If the fluid buildup is large, you may experience the following symptoms:

- Fullness or heaviness in the chest
- Discomfort or pain in the chest

Pleural space

The space between the membranes that line the inside of the chest wall and that cover the outside of the lungs.

Neurologic Problems, Fluid Retention, and Blood Chemistry

- Cough
- Shortness of breath

If you have these symptoms, discuss them with your doctor or nurse. The diagnosis of a pleural effusion is made by physical examination and chest x-ray. First, you will have a standing chest x-ray. Then you will be asked to lie down on your side (with the side with the fluid on the x-ray table), and another x-ray will be taken in this position. This is called a *lateral decubitus x-ray*. Pleural fluid can also be seen on a CT scan.

Treatment for pleural effusion depends on the amount of fluid in your chest and whether you are having related symptoms.

- If you have a small or medium pleural effusion that is not causing any symptoms, your doctor may recommend chemotherapy that will treat the tumor and make the fluid go away.
- If you have a large pleural effusion and shortness of breath or pain, the doctor can remove the fluid by means of a **thoracentesis**, that is, the removal of fluid from the pleural cavity through a needle inserted between the ribs. You do not need to be admitted to the hospital for this procedure.
- If the fluid comes back, your doctor may recommend **pleurodesis**, a medical procedure that uses chemicals or drugs to cause inflammation and adhesion between the layers of the pleura to prevent the buildup of fluid in the pleural cavity. The procedure, which is done in the hospital, begins with the insertion of a chest tube through the ribs into the pleural space and draining it dry. Once the fluid is removed, your doctor pushes a special medicine through the

Thoracentesis

Removal of fluid from the pleural cavity through a needle inserted between the ribs.

Pleurodesis

A medical procedure that uses chemicals or drugs to cause inflammation and adhesion between the layers of the pleura to prevent the buildup of fluid in the pleural cavity.

chest tube into the pleural space. The medicine causes irritation of the pleura and scar tissue to form. Once this happens, the pleura stick together, leaving no space for fluid to accumulate; for most people this permanently prevents fluid from building up again in the pleural space.

- Another option for the drainage of pleural effusions does not require a hospital stay. A thin tube, called a PleurX® Pleural Catheter, is inserted into your chest to drain fluid. You or a family member will be taught how to drain fluid from your chest while you are at home, and a visiting nurse can come into the home to help you with this. In many cases, the catheter can be removed within 30 days, and pleurodesis can be achieved without inserting any medicine into your chest. Ask your doctor if this procedure is an option for you.

If you have symptoms from a pleural effusion, you can do several things to make yourself more comfortable. If you have shortness of breath or if your breathing is difficult, your doctor may prescribe oxygen and medicine to make breathing easier, and sleeping on pillows or in a recliner may make breathing easier (see Question 46 for more information on management of shortness of breath). If you have pain, take your pain medicine as your doctor recommends.

79. My doctor has told me my blood chemistry can be affected by treatment. What does this mean?

A number of tests analyze the chemicals in your blood. Blood chemistry tests include the measurement of lipids, glucose (sugar), electrolytes, enzymes, vitamins, and hormones. Certain blood chemistry tests can tell us how

Neurologic Problems, Fluid Retention, and Blood Chemistry

well your organs are functioning. For example, liver function studies tell us how well your liver is working, and other studies tell us how well your kidneys, heart, and lungs are working. A blood chemistry test is similar to a complete blood count (CBC), which tells us how well your bone marrow (which makes blood cells) is working (see Question 35 for more information on blood counts).

Certain drugs used for cancer treatment depend on specific organs, such as the liver or kidneys, to be eliminated from the body. If these organs do not function normally, the drug levels can build up in your body and cause serious side effects.

Some treatments can damage specific organs in your body. Your doctor and nurse will do everything they can to prevent this from happening. For some treatments, they will give you large amounts of fluid intravenously or medicines before or after treatment to prevent organ damage. They may also instruct you to increase the amount of fluid you drink before or after treatment. You should take your medicine and drink fluid exactly as your doctor prescribes. You may even be asked to measure the amount of fluid that you drink and measure the amount of urine that you put out every day. If you are getting any treatment that can damage your organs, your doctor will measure your blood chemistry before you start treatment and then regularly while you are receiving treatment to be sure there is no damage and that the treatment is safe. If the blood tests show that any of your organs are not functioning normally, the doctor may decide to reduce the dose of the treatment or stop it altogether.

Some treatments can cause changes in your body chemicals, such as a lowered magnesium level in the blood. Blood chemistries can also be affected by dehydration, which may be caused by nausea, vomiting, or diarrhea. If you are suspected of having any of these problems, your doctor will also order blood chemistry tests. If the blood tests show that certain electrolytes are too low, your doctor may decide to replace them. (**Electrolytes** are chemicals [e.g., sodium, potassium, chloride, and calcium] in the blood that help regulate nerve and muscle function and help the body maintain its balance of fluid.) If the tests show you are dehydrated, you may be given extra intravenous fluids.

Sometimes people experience symptoms such as confusion or difficulty thinking, sleepiness, fatigue, nausea, or vomiting for reasons not related to blood chemistry. However, you should have all the tests your doctor orders because, most of the time, if you have the symptoms, your blood chemistry has been affected.

> Call your doctor or nurse if you have difficulty thinking, excessive sleepiness, or uncontrolled nausea, vomiting, or diarrhea.

80. I have heard that some people can get diabetes from their treatment. How is this diagnosed and treated?

The pancreas secretes a hormone called *insulin* into the bloodstream. Insulin enables **glucose** (a type of sugar and the chief source of energy for living organisms) to be transported into your cells, giving you energy throughout the day. Normally, the pancreas adjusts the amount of insulin secreted based on what you eat and on your activity level. This keeps the level of glucose in your blood controlled at about 80 to 120 milligrams per deciliter (mg/dl). If your pancreas is not able to secrete an adequate amount of insulin or if your

Electrolytes

Chemicals (e.g., sodium, potassium, chloride, and calcium) in the blood that help regulate nerve and muscle function and help the body maintain its balance of fluid.

Glucose

A type of sugar and the chief source of energy for living organisms.

body becomes partially resistant to insulin, the glucose cannot enter the cells effectively. As a result, the level of glucose in your blood will rise, called **hyperglycemia**, or abnormally high blood sugar. Diabetes is persistent hyperglycemia.

Hyperglycemia
Abnormally high blood sugar.

Here are some factors that increase a patient's risk of developing diabetes:

- Cancer of the pancreas
- Treatment with steroids
- A family history of diabetes
- Obesity, especially with high blood pressure and abnormal blood lipid levels

Diabetes is diagnosed by a blood test.

Symptoms of diabetes are frequent urination, thirst, fatigue, blurred vision, and weight loss. Diabetes is diagnosed by a blood test; an elevated fasting blood glucose level indicates the presence of diabetes.

Endocrinologist
A doctor who specializes in diagnosing and treating hormone disorders, including diabetes.

Throughout your treatment, your doctor will periodically check your blood chemistries, including the glucose level. If you develop persistent elevations in your blood glucose, you may be referred to an **endocrinologist**, a doctor who specializes in diagnosing and treating hormone disorders, including diabetes. Additional blood tests may be ordered, and the best treatment for you will be determined, which may involve a change in diet and an increase in exercise. You may also have to take either oral medication or insulin, which is injected under the skin. The endocrinologist may also arrange to have someone teach you how to test your blood glucose levels at home.

The goal of treatment is to keep your blood glucose levels as close to the normal range as possible. This goal is important to prevent long-term complications, which can result in heart and blood vessel disease, strokes, visual problems, kidney problems, and neurologic problems.

Additional information on diabetes is available from the National Diabetes Information Clearinghouse (www.diabetes.niddk.nih.gov).

81. What are paraneoplastic syndromes?

Paraneoplastic syndromes are believed to be caused by hormones or other substances that some tumors produce, causing symptoms in areas of the body at a distance from the tumor. For some people, a paraneoplastic syndrome can be the first sign leading to a diagnosis of cancer.

Paraneoplastic syndromes are rare. They occur more commonly in association with solid tumors, especially lung cancer, but they can occur with any cancer. Because these syndromes are caused by a tumor, treatment and control of the tumor usually result in their control too.

The usual signs and symptoms of a paraneoplastic syndrome are changes in the blood chemistry (e.g., high calcium, low sodium), peripheral neuropathy, joint pains, and an increased risk for blood clots. The diagnosis is made by physical examination, blood tests, x-ray, or ultrasound. The successful treatment of the cancer usually controls the paraneoplastic syndrome, but sometimes the doctor needs to give you additional medicine to treat the problem. You must take the medicine exactly as your doctor prescribes.

Neurologic Problems, Fluid Retention, and Blood Chemistry

PART EIGHT

Other Health-Related Issues

I get a flu shot every year.
Should I get one now that I am getting treated for
cancer?

Can I drink alcohol?

Should I stop smoking?

More . . .

82. I get a flu shot every year. Should I get one now that I am getting treated for cancer?

Pete's comment:

I have been getting the flu shot every year. In my case, the flu shot and pneumonia shot were administered by my oncologist. My wife also received both of these vaccinations to minimize the threat of her getting the flu and passing it on to me.

If you are getting treatment for cancer, get a flu shot every year. Influenza is a serious disease that occurs annually. If you get influenza while you are being treated for cancer, it is more difficult for your body to fight the virus and you can get very sick.

Influenza (flu) is a contagious virus that occurs every year; the peak season is usually from January through March. The most common symptoms of flu are fever, chills, cough, headache, muscle aches, and sore throat. If you get the flu, you will be sick for several days, and people who have weakened immune systems may get sicker and need to be hospitalized. Even if you get the flu shot, you can still catch the flu, but getting the shot reduces your chances of getting it, as well as the symptoms if you do get it.

The best time to get the flu shot is in October or November; however, you benefit from the shot even if you get it as late as January. You will be protected from the flu about 2 weeks after you get the shot, and this protection can last for as long as 1 year. Other members of your family should also get the flu shot to lessen their chances of getting the flu and giving it to you. Pregnant family members should check with their obstetrician before getting a flu shot.

The flu shot will not give you the flu, but it can cause some mild symptoms in the form of muscle aches and fever. Soreness, redness, or swelling at the injection may develop. Also, very rare symptoms of the flu shot are allergic reaction and Guillain-Barré syndrome. You should not take the flu shot if you are allergic to eggs, have a history of Guillain-Barré syndrome, or have had an allergic reaction to a previous flu shot. If you are sick or have a fever when the shot is scheduled, your doctor will postpone the injection until you recover. Your doctor may also decide to postpone your vaccination if your white blood cell count is low.

There are two types of influenza vaccine. The one that has been used for many years is the so-called "flu shot"; this is an inactivated (killed) form of the influenza virus. FluMist is a new way to get vaccinated for the flu; it is an intranasal, live, influenza vaccine. This vaccine is approved only for healthy people of ages 5 to 49.

> **If you are getting treatment for cancer, you and your family (or other household) members should *not* take FluMist.**

For more information about the flu shot, you can contact the Centers for Disease Control and Prevention (800-CDC-INFO [800-232-4636]) or on the Internet (www.cdc.gov/flu). You can also get information from your local or state health department.

83. What is the pneumonia vaccine? Should I get it?

Streptococcus pneumoniae is the bacteria that causes the most common kind of pneumonia in this country, pneumococcal pneumonia. Pneumococcal pneumonia is a serious disease that causes high fever, cough, and stabbing chest pains. The pneumococcal vaccine (Pneu-movax) reduces your chances of getting this type of pneumonia but does not prevent pneumonias caused by viruses or by bacteria other than *S. pneumoniae.*

If you are getting treatment for cancer, ask your doctor if you should get the pneumococcal vaccine. If you are getting treatment for Hodgkin's disease or having a bone marrow transplant, the timing of these treat-ments with the administration of the pneumococcal vaccine is critical. Check with your doctor before get-ting the vaccine.

Unlike the flu shot, which is given yearly, the pneumo-coccal vaccine is given once, and some people need to be revaccinated after 5 years. If you have had the pneu-mococcal vaccine more than 5 years ago and you are getting treatment for cancer, ask your doctor if you need to have another shot.

The pneumococcal vaccine can be given at the same time as the flu shot, but it should be given in the opposite arm. Don't get the pneumococcal vaccine if you have a fever or feel sick; it can be postponed until you feel well. You should not get the vaccine if you have an allergy to any component of the vaccine. The most common reactions to the vaccine are:

- Soreness, redness, and swelling at the vaccine site
- Fever
- Muscle aches
- Malaise

For more information on the pneumococcal vaccine, contact the Centers for Disease Control and Preven-tion (800-CDC-INFO [800-232-4636]), or you can

get information on the Internet (www.cdc.gov/
vaccines). You can also get information from your local
or state health department.

84. Is it safe for me to be around children who have recently received a vaccine?

In the United States, the Centers for Disease Control
and Prevention (CDC) recommends a regular schedule of vaccinations for children and adolescents. The
vaccination schedule starts at birth and goes up to the
ages of 13 to 18 years. The recommended vaccinations
include:

- Hepatitis A and B
- Diphtheria, tetanus, pertussis (DPT)
- Inactivated polio (a shot)
- Measles, mumps, rubella (MMR)
- Varicella (chickenpox)
- Influenza and pneumococcal vaccine (see Questions
  82 and 83)

All these are inactivated (killed) vaccines, except for
varicella and FluMist (the new inhaled influenza vaccine), which are "live" vaccines, made from weakened
viruses. Although rare, children (or adults) given the
varicella vaccine or FluMist could transmit the disease
to susceptible people.

If you are getting treatment for cancer and a member
of your household has been vaccinated, check with
your doctor or nurse to see if you should avoid contact
with the vaccinated person.

For more information, you can also contact the Centers
for Disease Control and Prevention (800-CDC-INFO
[800-232-4636]), or you can get information on the

Internet (www.cdc.gov/vaccines). You can also get information from your local or state health department.

85. Should I follow up with my regular doctors while I am getting treated for cancer?

If you are getting treatment for cancer, you should talk to your doctor or nurse about your regular health maintenance and disease prevention routines (e.g., mammogram, colonoscopy, dental care, Pap smear, PSA level, blood lipid level). You should continue your normal routine if possible, but, while you are getting your cancer therapy, some of these routines need to be scheduled at a "safe" time. Your other physicians need to be told that you have cancer and what treatment you are taking. For example, before making an appointment for dental work, notify your oncologist and your dentist. Together, they can decide when you should schedule your visit and if you need to take antibiotics or have a complete blood count before your appointment.

If you are getting treated for cancer, the doctor taking care of you is likely a medical, surgical, or radiation oncologist (a doctor who in the last few years of professional training specialized in the care of people with cancer). In addition to treating your cancer, an oncologist is capable of performing a complete history and physical examination, ordering and interpreting the results of tests, and prescribing medications. Make sure that your oncologist shares results of his or her examinations, tests, and prescriptions with your other doctors because doing so may cut down on the duplication of tests and extra expense for you and your insurance company.

Many people who have cancer also have other medical problems, such as diabetes, hypertension (high blood pressure), heart disease, lung disease, and arthritis. In some cases, if your medical problem is mild or well controlled, your oncologist may be able to help you manage or monitor it. In other circumstances, such as if you have difficulty controlling diabetes or heart disease, you should continue to see your personal physician. There is no right way to handle these circumstances. You and your oncologist need to make the decision together, depending on the seriousness of your cancer and your other health-related problems.

86. Can I drink alcohol?

Lisa's comment:

I was surprised when my nurse told me there were no alcohol restrictions during chemotherapy treatment for breast cancer. However, since most of my oncology nursing experience comes from the gastrointestinal service [esophageal, stomach, colon, rectal, liver, and pancreatic cancers], I couldn't help but refrain from alcohol consumption. If I drank at all, it was at least a week after treatment. I had few side effects during therapy. Perhaps not drinking was key?

Recently, much media attention has been directed to the health benefits of regular light to moderate alcohol consumption, with reports of a decreased incidence of stroke, positive effects on the heart, and other beneficial effects. Additionally, for many people, having a drink before dinner stimulates the appetite.

Alcohol can interact with many medications, including certain treatments for cancer, possibly resulting in intensifying the effects of some medications or making others ineffective. Additionally, even though alcohol is high in calories, high alcohol consumption can interfere with the absorption of nutrients in the stomach and small intestine. Furthermore, some antibiotics can cause severe nausea, vomiting, and headache when alcohol is consumed.

If you are getting treatment for cancer, talk to your doctor or nurse about consumption of alcohol while you are getting treatment. Depending on your circumstances, you may be able to have an occasional drink. Other doctors will recommend that you do not drink any alcohol at all.

87. Should I stop smoking?

There are no benefits to smoking tobacco products. Smoking contributes to serious respiratory diseases (emphysema and chronic bronchitis), peripheral vascular disease (diseases of the blood vessels that carry blood to the arms and legs), and heart disease. In addition to causing lung cancer, smoking is also a risk factor for other cancers of the mouth (oral), voice box (larynx), bladder, kidney, pancreas, cervix, and stomach, and for some types of leukemia.

> There are no benefits to smoking tobacco. If you continue to smoke, you are at greater risk for side effects of surgery, chemotherapy, and radiation therapy.

If you have cancer or are getting treatment for cancer, stop smoking. Research has shown that people with cancer who stop smoking live longer than those who do not, even in people who have lung cancer. If you continue to smoke, you are at increased risk for side effects of surgery, chemotherapy, and radiation therapy. You are also at increased risk of developing a second type of cancer. Smoking also increases the risk of developing other diseases.

Some people have little or no difficulty when they stop smoking; others are either unable to quit or they resume smoking later. Some people are nicotine dependent and can experience withdrawal symptoms when they stop smoking. If you are currently smoking tobacco products, talk to your doctor or nurse, who can recommend strategies for quitting.

Nicotine replacement therapy, other medicines, behavioral modification, and support groups are available to help you quit smoking, and a combination of all these elements is used in comprehensive smoking cessation programs. Your doctor or nurse can recommend a program for you.

There are a number of nicotine replacement therapies. Nicotine gum and nicotine patch (Nicorette, Habitrol, NicoDerm CQ) are available over the counter. Nicotine inhaler and nicotine spray (Nicotrol) are available by prescription. All nicotine replacement products are associated with side effects, such as:

- Headache
- Dizziness
- Upset stomach
- Blurred vision
- Unusual dreams or nightmares
- Diarrhea

People who have significant heart problems, including a recent heart attack, should use nicotine replacement therapy with caution. To see if nicotine replacement therapy is safe for you, check with your doctor or nurse.

Bupropion (Zyban) and varenicline (Chantix), available by prescription, can help you quit smoking and reduce withdrawal symptoms. Bupropion was originally used as an antidepressant (called Wellbutrin), but

Other Health-Related Issues

research shows that this medicine is also helpful for people who want to quit smoking. These medicines, used alone, are often not enough to make people quit smoking. Bupropion is typically used in addition to nicotine replacement therapy as part of a smoking cessation program. Chantix is not used with other medications, but support groups or behavioral modification may be used to help you quit smoking.

For more information on smoking cessation, you can call the American Cancer Society (800-227-2345) or go online (www.cancer.org, search "kick the habit"). Additional information on smoking cessation and nicotine replacement therapy can be obtained through the American Lung Association (800-586-4872, www.lungusa.org, search "quit smoking"). Quitnet (www.quitnet.com) is an online program that is available to help people quit smoking; many have found this site to be informative and helpful.

PART NINE

Emotional and Social Concerns

How can I better cope with having cancer?

How do I go on with my life and start feeling "normal" again?

How can I talk with family and friends about my cancer?

More . . .

88. How can I better cope with having cancer?

Lisa's comment:

My ability to cope with the diagnosis of cancer probably stems from having a strong oncology knowledge base. I think I would have been more overwhelmed if I didn't know anything about cancer and its treatments. It is true, though, that too much knowledge can be a bad thing!

I'm a no-nonsense type of gal. Once diagnosed, I sought the best medical care possible, had confidence in my physicians and nurses, and accepted the love and support of family and friends. I received comfort in my already active religious life and truly felt my burdens spiritually lifted.

Pete's comment:

The emotions that I went through after being told that I have lung cancer ran the gamut from anger to fear to emotional overload. I had thought of myself as a relatively healthy man who was in good physical condition. Now, I face a devastating cancer diagnosis that could dramatically affect my quality of life. I was also dejected and frustrated that I would not be able to accomplish so many things that I wanted to do. I find that by focusing on the moment and the "next right thing," I am able to keep things in perspective and prevent myself from getting out of control. I also find that by discussing options, approaches, and priorities constantly with my wife, I am able to feel much more comfortable.

When confronted with any type of difficulty or stressful situation, people tend to react and cope in ways that are characteristic for them. Some people tend to turn away from what is happening and try to shut it out for a while, whereas others tend to face things head-on. Some people are comfortable facing difficulties alone, whereas others prefer to have the support of family or friends. Some people want to share their thoughts and feelings about the experience, and others are more private and prefer not to talk about how they are feeling. Some people use humor to help them face difficulties; the approach of others is much more serious. Some people want detailed information about what is happening, whereas others want to hear only what they must know. Some people want to be actively involved in making all the decisions that must be made, and others prefer to defer the decision making to their family or to their doctor.

How have you generally responded to difficulties or solved problems in your life? What strategies do you characteristically use when faced with stressful situations? Have these worked for you in the past? Do you feel they will be effective for you in facing the challenges ahead of you now? If you feel comfortable with the coping strategies you have used in the past and feel confident that they will be effective for you now, there is no reason to think you have to change. In fact, it is helpful to explain to your family, friends, doctors, and nurses what coping strategies are most effective for you so they that can support you in using these.

However, if you feel that your typical ways of coping may not be effective in dealing with your cancer, or if you feel the challenges are too great, learning new ways of coping will help. You may be able to learn new ways of coping on your own or by speaking with family and friends, but many people find it helpful to work with a professional counselor or therapist. Question 91 has suggestions on how to find professional help.

89. I feel so many different emotions throughout the day. How can I feel more in control?

When faced with a life-threatening illness, you may react with many different emotions. You may find yourself denying the diagnosis at times and having difficulty acknowledging or accepting the full reality of what you are facing. You may feel anger that all this is happening to you, anger at the medical establishment, anger at yourself, or even anger at God. You may feel worried about what treatment will be like and about your uncertain future. You may feel sad about the disruptions in your life, the loss of your independence, or the possible loss of the future you had planned. Most people with cancer experience some or all of these feelings at one time or another. You can expect these feelings to be especially strong at certain times. The difficult times, for many people, are when they are first told of the diagnosis, when they are faced with making decisions, just before they start treatment, when they find out the cancer has recurred or spread, or when they find their cancer no longer has an effective treatment. At these times, do not be surprised if feelings that you thought had passed earlier come back to the surface.

There is no right or wrong way to feel. Try to put your thoughts and feelings into words so that you can better understand what you are experiencing.

There is no right or wrong way to feel. Trying to block your feelings or to control them may cause you undue distress or suffering. Instead, put your thoughts and feelings into words so that you can better understand what you are experiencing. You can do this in a number of ways, and a combination of strategies may work best for you:

- Reflect on your experience; try to clarify in your mind what you are thinking and feeling.

- Write your thoughts and feelings in a journal.
- Talk about your thoughts and feelings with someone you trust and feel supported by. This person can be a close family member or friend, your doctor or nurse, a professional counselor or therapist, or a religious leader or pastoral counselor. Many people feel an immediate sense of relief once they have said out loud what they are feeling inside.
- Talk with other cancer patients and listen to how they describe their experiences.

Regardless of your approach, once you have recognized exactly what your thoughts and feelings are, you will be better able to clarify what you want and need. You can then direct your energy to getting these needs met, and you will feel more in control.

You can use other strategies to improve how you feel emotionally. Many people find that physical activity, even a brief walk or bike ride, enhances their feeling of well-being. Others make use of specific mind–body techniques, such as progressive muscle relaxation (alternately tensing and relaxing the muscles in one part of the body at a time), hypnosis, meditation, and mental imagery.

90. Are there support groups where I can talk with other patients going through the same thing as I am?

Support groups provide the opportunity to be with other cancer patients. You can share your thoughts and feelings with the group, and you can hear how other people have reacted to and dealt with the same challenges you are facing. Groups can be very helpful because one of the most difficult parts of having cancer

Many people feel an immediate sense of relief once they have said out loud what they are feeling inside.

Emotional and Social Concerns

is feeling alone—that no one really understands what you are going through.

Think about what type of group would be most helpful to you when making your selection. A health professional or a trained patient leader generally leads a support group. Groups may be set up only for people with a particular kind of cancer, or they may be open to people with any type of cancer. They may be very structured, or they may be social and informal. They may be very educationally focused, with speakers on different topics, or they may provide interaction and sharing of people's individual experiences. They may be just for patients, just for families, or for both. They may meet for a defined period of time with a limited membership, or they may be open-ended, allowing people to come and go as they like.

There are increasing numbers of online support groups, chat rooms, and e-mail discussion groups, some of them for patients with a particular type of cancer. Keep in mind that online support groups are usually not moderated by a professional, and the information you receive may not be accurate. If you get recommendations or advice from an online support group, discuss them with your doctor.

There are a number of ways to find out about support groups where you live or on the Internet. Ask your doctor or nurse to direct you to a group or call the Department of Social Work at your local hospital. Other resources are:

- *American Cancer Society:* www.cancer.org or 800-ACS-2345
- *Cancer Care:* www.cancercare.org or 800-813-HOPE

- *Gilda's Club:* www.gildasclub.org or 888-GILDA-4-U
- *The Wellness Community:* www.thewellnesscommunity. org or 888-793-WELL
- *OncoChat:* www.oncochat.org
- *Cancer Hope Network:* www.cancerhopenetwork.org or 877-467-3638 (This site provides one-on-one support by matching patients with trained volunteers who have received a similar diagnosis and who have gone through treatment and recovered.)
- *Association of Cancer Online Resources:* www.acor.org

91. My emotions are often overwhelming, and I feel distressed much of the time. How do I know if I need professional help? Where can I get professional help in coping with my emotional concerns or to improve my ability to cope with having cancer?

As described in Question 89, reacting with many different emotions after being diagnosed with cancer is normal. Try to differentiate these normal emotional reactions from those that may be causing you significant distress or suffering. Here are some signs that you are in distress:

- You are having so much difficulty accepting the reality of what is happening to you that you cannot make decisions about your care.
- You are so angry that you are not able to trust your health care providers.
- You are so worried and anxious that you find it difficult to understand and absorb the information you are getting, to make decisions, or to solve everyday problems.
- You feel anxious much of the time, with an ongoing feeling that something dreadful is going to happen.

Emotional and Social Concerns

Psychiatrists

Doctors who specialize in the prevention, diagnosis, and treatment of mental illness; a psychiatrist can prescribe medicine.

Psychologists

Specialists who can talk with patients and their families about emotional and personal matters and who can help them make decisions.

Psychiatric nurses

Registered nurses who care for patients with mental health issues; some provide counseling; nurse practitioners have advanced degrees and can prescribe medication.

Social workers

Professionals who are trained to talk with people and their families about emotional or physical needs and to find them support services.

You may also feel nervous, shaky, or jittery; sweat; feel tightness in your chest or stomach; or feel that your heart is racing.

- You are sad and tearful throughout most of the day.
- You have become depressed and lost interest or pleasure in aspects of your life that you previously enjoyed. This may be accompanied by feelings of despair or hopelessness or by problems with energy, sleep, appetite, or concentration.
- You find yourself unable to communicate as you usually do with your family or friends.

If you are experiencing any of these continuously for more than 2 weeks, or if your feelings become very upsetting or interfere with your daily life, discuss the symptoms with your doctor or nurse. Although your feelings may not seem important enough to discuss with your doctor, addressing emotional distress is as important as addressing physical symptoms you may have. Ask your doctor or nurse about obtaining help from a mental health professional. Seeking this kind of treatment is not a sign of weakness, and in fact can enhance your ability to cope, particularly if you have had anxiety or depression in the past. Treatment can involve therapeutic counseling and medication, as well as a variety of techniques using your body and mind.

Many types of professionals can help you deal with your emotions and improve your ability to cope with having cancer. **Psychiatrists, psychologists, psychiatric nurses,** and **social workers** are all licensed or certified in their specialties and can all provide counseling. In addition, psychiatrists can prescribe medicine and social workers can help find support services. Religious leaders, pastoral counselors, or hospital chaplains can also assist you to find strength and support in the spiritual dimension of your life.

You can get referrals to one of these professionals in a number of ways:

- Ask your doctor or nurse.
- Contact your hospital's Department of Social Work, Department of Psychiatry, or Chaplaincy Service.
- Contact Cancer Care, the American Cancer Society, or the Cancer Information Service of the National Cancer Institute.
- Speak with the religious leader at your local house of worship.

92. I have completed treatment and my doctor tells me there is no evidence of cancer. How do I go on with my life and start feeling "normal" again?

Lisa's comment:

I never felt so loved before than when being diagnosed with cancer. I received well wishes, telephone calls, visits, flowers, get-well cards, and mass cards from everyone in various aspects of my life. And, yes, my relationship with family and friends has been enhanced and enriched. I didn't think it was possible.

Completing treatment for cancer brings its own set of challenges. Among these are adjusting to changes in your body, recovering strength after treatment, resuming your usual activities, returning to work, and explaining your illness to friends and colleagues. Each of these presents a new hurdle to overcome. Give yourself time and remember to draw on your usual methods of coping as well as those that are newly learned as you transition into feeling "normal" again (see Question 88).

Despite the fact that your treatment is over, you will probably find it difficult at times to balance the hopefulness that the disease will not come back with the knowledge that the future is always uncertain. Maintain a schedule of regular follow-up visits with your doctor, who will schedule blood tests and scans periodically to evaluate how you are doing. Many people find that the days immediately before their doctor's appointments and the days waiting for the results of diagnostic tests are times of anxiety and worry.

Advances in treatment in recent years have led to increasing numbers of cancer survivors and increasing resources to address their needs. A number of resources may be helpful to you as you adjust to your life as a cancer survivor. The following resources provide practical suggestions on specific topics, describe the experiences of other survivors, provide the opportunity to interact with other survivors, and list links to other resources:

- *Facing Forward: Life after Cancer Treatment* (published by the National Cancer Institute): www.cancer.gov or 800-4-CANCER
- *Lance Armstrong Foundation:* www.livestrong.org or 866-673-7205
- *Cancer Survivors Network of the American Cancer Center:* www.csn.cancer.org
- *National Coalition for Cancer Survivorship:* www.canceradvocacy.org or 888-650-9127

Despite the fears and uncertainties that lie ahead, some people find that having been diagnosed with cancer has provided them the opportunity to think about their lives in new ways. Relationships often become stronger and are enriched by the experience.

And sometimes people choose to shift the priorities in their life, ensuring they are spending their time doing what is most important to them.

DEALING WITH FRIENDS, FAMILY, AND WORK

93. How can I talk with family and friends about my cancer?

Lisa's comment:

During the early stages of my diagnosis and surgical plans, I remember getting fed up repeating myself to various friends or talking incessantly about my treatment plan or cancer in general. I would finally say, "Could we please change the subject!" I am not one to dwell on things or to be fussed over, and cancer did not change that aspect of my personality!

For some people, having cancer is a lonely experience. However, for others it is a time of feeling closely connected with friends and family. Being able to talk with others about your cancer can make an enormous difference in how you experience this challenging time in your life. It can help to overcome the feeling that you are alone, and it provides others the opportunity to offer you their help and support. However, you may not be ready to share your thoughts and feelings right away, and over time you may want to share some feelings but keep others private. Decide what you want to share about your diagnosis, treatment, and prognosis.

If family or friends are pressuring you to speak about this before you are ready, tell them that you appreciate their concern but that you are just not ready to talk yet. Don't push them away; reassure them that you will

Emotional and Social Concerns

speak with them when you are ready. You may find that some friends or family members pull away from you, not calling or visiting as they used to. This may be because they are sad or are afraid of saying the wrong thing and upsetting you. Consider how important this person is to you. If it is someone you don't care very much about, there is no reason to spend any time or energy trying to reach out. However, if you value your relationship with this person, you may want to call them and directly express to them that you miss them. Tell them that you wish you could speak to them or see them more often, and ask if there is anything you can do to make it easier for them. This may break the ice and allow them to feel more comfortable. Although some people will disappoint you, others will surprise you with their kindness, helpfulness, and desire to be present in your life to provide support.

94. How can I talk with children about my cancer?

A common reaction is to try to protect children from the news that a family member has cancer for fear of frightening or upsetting them. However, children can always sense when something is wrong at home. It is much better for them to hear directly from you about what is happening rather than overhearing something by accident or imagining the worst.

Children cope best when they are informed. Select language that is appropriate to their age and ability to understand.

Children cope best when they are informed. Set aside time to talk with them as soon as possible after you have been diagnosed and be open and honest when you speak with them. You may want to include the following information:

• The fact that you are sick and that you have cancer
• The type of treatment that is planned

- Whether you will need to be in the hospital for a while
- The likely side effects of treatment and how they will affect how you look and what you will be able to do

When speaking with children, select language that is appropriate to their age and ability to understand. You might find it helpful to practice what you want to say before you sit down with them. After you have spoken with them, encourage the children to ask questions, and check to see that they understand what you have told them. However, be aware that they may be able to hear only so much at a time. You may need to break down the information and address only one or two topics at a time when you speak with them.

Your children may ask if you will die, or they may ask for reassurance that you will get better. Respond to their questions as honestly as you can. If you have been diagnosed with cancer at an early stage with a high probability of cure, reassure them. However, if you have advanced disease and they ask if you will die, you might want to explain that some people die from cancer and that the doctor is not sure right now if they can make the cancer go away. Tell them that you are hoping you will be okay and that the doctor is doing everything possible to help you. If they ask when your treatment will be over, tell them the planned date if you will be receiving treatment for a defined period of time. However, it is okay to tell them you don't know. Reassure them that as things change you will tell them what is happening.

Describe to your children how your disease and treatment will affect them. Explain who will take care of them if you will be in the hospital or if you will be coming home late from doctor visits or treatments. Explain how their usual routines and activities may be affected. Be sure to ask them if there is anything in particular they are worried about.

A number of resources are available to help you speak with children about cancer and to help them cope with your diagnosis:

- *American Cancer Society:* www.cancer.org or 800-ACS-2345 (Search the site for the many resources available, including books for children.)
- *When Your Parent Has Cancer, a Guide for Teens* (published by the National Cancer Institute): www.cancer.gov or 800-4-CANCER
- *Helping Children When a Family Member Has Cancer* (published by Cancer Care): www.cancercare.org or 800-813-HOPE
- *KidsCope*: www.kidscope.org or 404-892-1437
- *Children's Treehouse Foundation*: childrenstreehousefdn.org or 303-322-1202 (See the books published by this group listed on the site.)
- *When a Parent Is Sick: Helping Parents Explain Serious Illness to Children*, by Joan Hamilton (published by Pottersfield Press and available through Nimbus Publishing at 800-646-2879 and Amazon.com)

95. Should I work during my treatment? Should I tell my supervisor and coworkers about my diagnosis? What if I don't feel well enough to work?

Lisa's comment:

- *I felt compelled to share my diagnosis with my colleagues almost immediately. I work in an oncology setting. I wanted to openly discuss my hopes and desires, fears and concerns. I felt my absence from work affected them, so they deserved to know why I would not be around for a while. I also didn't want my colleagues to feel like they couldn't talk to me about my disease and treatment. I didn't want to be uncomfortable with my life changes, and therefore they wouldn't be uncomfortable either. After surgery and my first cycle of chemotherapy, I returned to work. I felt a need for normalcy and I wanted to help with staffing. My supervisor and coworkers were tremendously supportive and truthfully helped me through the chemotherapy and radiation treatments.*

If you feel productive and energized by your work or if you enjoy the camaraderie you experience at work, you will probably want to continue working during your treatment if you are able. Many people feel quite well during cancer treatment and can continue working, either full-time or part-time. However, other people do not feel well enough to work or must make accommodations in their hours of work or in their specific functions. Tell your doctor or nurse about the type of work you do and your usual hours of work. Ask how you can expect to feel during treatment and if you will be able to continue working.

People who continue to work often feel unsure whether to tell anyone about their situation, whom to tell, and how much to tell. Some people want to talk openly about their diagnosis and treatment with colleagues, whose support helps them cope with treatment. Other people are more private and prefer that people at work not know about their situation. Some people are even afraid that, if people at work know they are ill, they will be treated differently, be discriminated against, or even lose their jobs.

The Americans with Disabilities Act protects disabled people from discrimination at work. It requires employers to make reasonable accommodations as long as you can perform the essential functions of your job. However, people unfortunately do not always respond as we hope they will or as the law requires. You may find that your supervisor believes you will not be able to perform as well on the job, and you may lose the opportunity to work on certain projects or even to be promoted. You may find that your coworkers will be uncomfortable hearing about your diagnosis. They may pull away from you, not interacting with you as they used to. This reaction may be because they are sad or afraid of saying the wrong thing and upsetting you. Some coworkers may worry that they will have to do more work because of your illness, which may make them resentful.

Speak with your supervisor or someone in the human resources department about your options.

If you need accommodations in the type of your work or in your hours, you must speak with your supervisor about the situation. Prepare ahead for this conversation. First, consider how you can get the most important parts of your job done. Then determine how you need to alter the hours you work to balance getting the job done with taking care of your medical needs. Being open with your supervisor from the beginning can be extremely helpful. A supervisor can guide you in obtaining information about your rights and your benefits, in addition to working with you to make the accommodations you need and to make adjustments over time as your needs change. If you find it difficult to speak directly with your supervisor about this, speak with someone in the human resources department. If you have a conflict with your supervisor and human resources is not able to help, you may need to contact an attorney for guidance.

You can contact the following organizations for more information about the Americans with Disabilities Act and how it applies to you:

- *United States Department of Justice:* www.ada.gov or 800-514-0301
- *United States Equal Employment Opportunity Commission:* www.eeoc.gov or 800-669-4000

If you are unable to work or must change to part-time work, speak with your supervisor or someone in the human resources department about your options. Find out about your disability benefits. Be aware that the Family and Medical Leave Act allows eligible employees up to a total of 12 weeks of unpaid leave during any 12-month period. For information about this, contact the human resources department where you work or the United States Department of Labor (www.dol.gov/esa/whd/fmla or 866-487-9243).

Cancer and Careers (www.cancerandcareers.org) is a valuable resource for people with cancer, their employers, and their coworkers. It addresses related issues and provides helpful tips and suggestions from other patients about living and working with cancer.

FOR FAMILY AND FRIENDS

96. How can I help? What is the right thing to say?

Knowing how best to help someone you care about who has been diagnosed with cancer is often difficult. No answer to this question is right for everyone. Consider what you are able to do and would like to do, and then try to match this with what the person needs.

You may find it easiest to start with concrete things. However, a general offer like "Let me know if I can help with anything" is often not the best approach. This type of offer requires the person to think about what he or she needs and then ask you for help. Instead, try to anticipate what the person will need and make specific offers. Plan these for days when you know the person may need more help than usual, like days of doctor visits or treatment or when the person is feeling ill or tired. The possibilities are unlimited, but here are a few examples of offers you might make:

*Try to antici-
pate what the
person will
need and make
specific offers.*

- Driving them to a doctor visit or treatment
- Dropping off a cooked dinner for the family
- Spending a morning cleaning the house
- Laundering the family clothes
- Shopping for food and needed household items
- Inviting the children for a sleepover
- Arranging to pick up or meet the children after school

Another way of helping is to offer your presence. Someone might appreciate company if living alone or while the rest of the family is working or at school. Offer to visit and bring lunch, to accompany the person for a walk, to bring a video you can both watch, to go out shopping together, or to spend the weekend with you. Again, the possibilities are unlimited. The key is to match what you are able to do and would like to do with the specific things the person enjoys.

A word of caution: Cancer patients may not have the energy to participate in many of the things you used to do together. Consider how they are feeling at the time, and don't create unrealistic expectations for them. You may need to plan short visits. Make the time together pleasurable regardless of what you do or how long a time you spend together.

It is natural to feel unsure of the right things to say when someone you care about has been diagnosed with cancer, is undergoing difficult treatment, or perhaps is facing the end of his or her life. You may feel afraid to ask cancer patients how they are doing because you are nervous you will not know how to respond to their answers. You may feel concerned that, if you say the wrong thing, you will hurt them. You may feel worried that, if you talk about your own sadness or even cry, you will cause the person distress. Because of your own discomfort, you may try to withdraw from the situation, distancing yourself from the person, calling less often, and putting off visits. This can result in leaving them feeling abandoned and alone at a time when they need your presence in their life more than ever before.

There is no script for what to say. In fact, if you make assumptions about what the person is thinking or feeling, you may unintentionally say things that will cause distress. The best way to start is by listening. Let it be known that you are ready to listen if the person wants to talk. At the same time, remember that not everyone communicates in the same way. Some people are very open and want to share everything they are thinking and feeling with those they are close to. Others are more private and prefer not to talk much. Even for people who are generally communicative, they may sometimes feel like talking and sometimes not. The important thing is to let the person control when and how much to share. If they want to speak with you of their thoughts and feelings, the greatest gift you can give is to be present and to listen.

The greatest gift you can give is to be present and to listen.

Emotional and Social Concerns

However, listening to things that are painful to hear about or being with someone who is emotionally distressed or crying may be uncomfortable for you. You may find yourself wanting to change the subject or even offering reassurances that everything will be okay, even if that may not necessarily be true. Although these reactions may help you deal with your own discomfort as the listener, they don't help the person speaking. In addition, they may send the message that you do not really want to hear what has to be said. Try to overcome your own discomfort and remain present to hear what the person is saying. It's okay to tell the person that this is difficult for you and that you are not sure how to respond to what you're hearing.

It's okay to tell the person that this is difficult for you and that you are not sure how to respond to what you're hearing.

You also may want to share your own thoughts or feelings. You may want to say how much you love and care about him or her. You may want to describe your own sadness or feelings of helplessness. You may want to try to reconcile if you've had a conflict. You may want to talk about your own worries and concerns related to the illness. We often leave a great deal unsaid in an attempt to protect those we love. Yet in fact it is the unsaid things that are often the most important things to say.

> *Caregiving for Your Loved One with Cancer* is available online (www.cancercare.org/pdf/booklets/ccc_caregiver.pdf).

97. At times I feel that the responsibility of caring for this person is very difficult. Do other people experience such feelings?

When someone is diagnosed with cancer, numerous stresses and demands are placed on family and friends. These stresses are influenced by how old the patient is, the role they play in the family, how advanced the disease is, the type of treatment they are getting, the symptoms they are experiencing, how physically disabled they are, and how they are emotionally responding to their illness. Regardless of individual situations, there are several sources of stress for those who are providing care.

One demand placed on caregivers is the need to provide physical care to the patient. The past 20 years have brought many changes in health care. One of the most significant is that many people who were previously cared for in the hospital are now cared for at home. This shift places the responsibility to provide physical care on family and friends: ensuring the person is comfortable; administering medications; managing equipment and supplies; observing for relevant signs or symptoms; knowing when to call the doctor or nurse; and, if the person is very ill, helping with bathing, dressing, feeding, moving, and walking. If the person has advanced disease, these demands increase if the person gets sicker.

Another demand placed on caregivers is the need to address the nonmedical aspects of care: scheduling and coordinating appointments, providing transportation, obtaining medications, running errands, supervising others who may be providing care, and handling medical bills and other financial matters. In addition, numerous decisions have to be made every day and problems regularly solved.

Making caregiving even more difficult is the fact that, when you become a caregiver, your usual day-to-day responsibilities don't just go away, and you may also have to take on responsibilities previously handled by the patient. Further complications arise when the caregiver, based on the previous relationship with the patient, may have ambivalent feelings about the fact that now he or she needs to take care of them.

All the stresses and demands placed on you as a caregiver can lead you to feel overwhelmed at times. You may become exhausted or even physically ill. In addition, you may find yourself experiencing a variety of difficult emotions: anger, guilt, fear, and sadness. Finding ways to care for yourself, attending to your physical and emotional needs, and using the available resources, can enable you to meet the needs of the patient and make the experience a positive and meaningful one for you. Question 98 lists resources available to help caregivers succeed in this role.

Finding ways to care for yourself can help you attend to the needs of the patient.

98. How can I get help so that I can provide support and care to this person without being overwhelmed by the demands?

The physical and emotional demands of caregiving are significant. The first step to getting help is to acknowledge how this is affecting you and to identify which demands are the greatest for you.

- Are you having difficulty in regard to the *time* needed for care: visiting in the hospital, accompanying the person to doctor visits or treatment, having to do more at home, or needing to take time off from work?
- Are you having difficulty in regard to the *finances* needed for care: inadequate medical insurance for doctor visits and treatments, expensive medications, costs of travel, costs of missed work time, and costs

of extra services you need to pay for, like extra babysitting?

- Are you having difficulty in regard to the *physical burdens* of providing care if the person is weak and debilitated: needing to assist with walking or lifting, needing to bathe and feed, needing to administer medications, perhaps needing to move in with the patient for a period of time?
- Are you having difficulty with the overall responsibility of *managing the medical care* when you don't feel you have adequate knowledge or skills to do this effectively?

You can take several approaches to manage the demands placed on you as a caregiver. The most important is to ensure that you have the information you need to feel capable of providing care. Schedule time to speak with the person's doctor or nurse in the office or over the phone to review the plan of care and discuss issues of concern to you. Here are some specific questions you may want to ask:

- What is the goal of treatment?
- What do you expect will be the outcome of the treatment?
- What side effects may occur from the treatment?
- How can the side effects be managed?
- What medications have been prescribed? What are they for? What dose should be given and at what times of the day?
- What are reasons I should call your office?

Ask for any written material that reinforces the information they have reviewed with you.

To manage the many things that must be done each day, divide the work. See if family members and

To manage the many things that must be done each day, divide the work.

friends are able and willing to do some part of the work. However, remember that people do not always respond as you want them to respond. Families that generally work well together in times of stress will work well together in providing care. However, families with a previous history of disagreement may find it difficult to overcome patterns of conflict. Furthermore, various members of the family will have different ideas about what they can manage, and their abilities may not match your expectations. Based on the various members' abilities and willingness, assign a schedule for them to do the tasks needed.

If you need more assistance at home than family or friends can provide, ask your doctor or nurse for a referral to a social worker to explore the possibility of home care services. These services include visits by:

- A registered nurse to provide skilled nursing care (e.g., changing a dressing, giving an injection)
- A home health aide to assist with personal care (e.g., bathing or being present in the home to assist the person during the hours you are not available)
- Homemakers to assist with tasks at home (e.g., cooking, cleaning, and laundry)

You will need to verify with the person's health insurance company what services are covered. If there is no coverage for help at home, consider approaching other members of the family who have the financial resources to pay for these services.

Other resources may be helpful in providing support to you as a caregiver. Educational programs designed specifically for caregivers of cancer patients may be available in your community. You can find out about them through the American Cancer Society, the Cancer Information Service of the National Cancer Institute, Cancer Care, or the department of social work at your local hospital. Here are some other good resources:

- *National Family Caregivers Association:* www.nfcacares.org or 800-896-3650
- *National Coalition for Cancer Survivorship:* cancer-advocacy.org (The Cancer Survival Toolbox includes a section entitled "Caring for the Caregiver.")
- *National Caregivers Library:* www.caregiverslibrary.org
- *Caregiving: A Step-by-Step Resource for Caring for the Person with Cancer at Home* (published by the American Cancer Society)

Key to being able to provide care is to find ways of taking care of your own needs. Combat the isolation many caregivers feel by reaching out to people who can support you. Spend time with them, and talk about how things are going. Schedule time for yourself to do things you enjoy, like taking a walk, listening to music, or reading a book. Don't try to do everything yourself; divide the work and let others help.

Combat the isolation many caregivers feel by reaching out to people who can support you.

Caregiving is stressful and brings many demands. It can be seen as a burden or as an opportunity. In caring for another person, you may learn of inner strengths that you never knew you had, you may find you are more competent and capable than you had previously realized, and you may feel spiritually enriched. Family and friends may come together with a renewed sense of purpose and connection. And finally, caregiving provides you the opportunity to express your love for the person in the most intimate way imaginable.

Emotional and Social Concerns

99. How do we manage the financial burdens that cancer places on our family?

When a person is diagnosed and treated for cancer, the financial burdens placed on the family are enormous. The patient may not be able to deal with the many financial issues that must be addressed; so many people find it helpful if a particular family member or friend takes over the responsibility. A number of steps are helpful in this situation.

Review the patient's health care benefits thoroughly to determine exactly what is covered. Many policies are confusing, and, if you are not clear on the benefits, speak with someone in the human resources department where the person works or contact the insurance company directly. Here are specific questions you may want to ask:

- Can any doctor treat the person, or must you use someone in the health plan? How much more will you have to pay to use a doctor outside the plan (*out of network*)?
- Does the plan include coverage for a second opinion?
- Is authorization needed before having particular diagnostic tests or treatments? What is the process for obtaining authorization?
- Does the plan cover care only at particular hospitals?
- Does the plan provide home care only with particular agencies?
- Does the plan include coverage for prescription medications?

Meet with a financial counselor where the person will be receiving treatment to determine the estimated costs of care. Work with the counselor to calculate what you have to pay out of pocket based on the insurance coverage. If you will not be able to pay the estimated amount, discuss how you can work out a realistic payment plan.

If paying for care will be difficult, meet with a social worker to find out what financial assistance is available. The person may be entitled to government or charitable assistance. The American Cancer Society and Cancer Care may also be able to provide financial assistance. An excellent resource on financial issues can be found at the American Society of Clinical Oncology (www.cancer.net/managingcostofcare). The section on "Financial Resources" lists many possibilities for obtaining financial assistance.

The cost of prescription medications can be significant. Many pharmaceutical companies have assistance programs to provide medication at a reduced cost. To find out about financial assistance available for particular medications, ask the nurse or social worker for information. A helpful resource that specifically addresses financial assistance for medications is NeedyMeds (www.needymeds.org).

Transportation is another area in which the financial costs can quickly mount. Speak with a social worker to get information about transportation services in the region. Cancer Care and the American Cancer Society can also provide information and may be able to offer limited financial assistance for transportation.

Track all the financial costs incurred related to the disease and treatment. When the person is first diagnosed, speak with an accountant to learn what is tax deductible and what records you should keep. The following costs are tax deductible for many people:

- *Medical costs not covered by insurance:* These include annual deductible costs, copays (the fees paid up front for specific services), and coinsurance (the part of the bill the insurance company doesn't cover). Keep copies of all bills and claim forms.
- *Expenses paid to maintain the person's health insurance policy.*
- *Out-of-pocket expenses:* These are expenses paid for prescription medications and transportation to medical appointments. Keep mileage records and receipts for all of these.

100. Where can I get more information about cancer symptoms and side effects of treatment?

The Internet is increasingly becoming the most up-to-date source of comprehensive information on cancer and cancer treatment. If you do not have a computer of your own, ask family members or friends if you can spend time using theirs. Most local libraries also have computers available to use for free, and hospitals are increasingly making computers available for patients and families to use.

Most of the Internet addresses we have listed in the appendix that follows will bring you to the home page of each organization. Although specific areas of the site may be pointed out, spend time searching within each site to find the information you are looking for, as well as to explore the other information and links. Your time will be rewarded as you increase your knowledge and understanding of the disease and treatment and as you discover the numerous resources for information and support that are available to help you, your family, and friends.

Tips for managing cancer symptoms and the side effects of treatment are found on many of these sites. Additional sites are mentioned within questions addressing particular symptoms or side effects. However, we urge you to speak with your doctor or nurse before trying anything recommended on the Internet.

Internet addresses often change over time. Those listed in the appendix are all accurate as of December 2009. If you cannot find the organization at the address listed, try using a **search engine** to find it. Telephone numbers are also listed if they are available.

Search engine

A service on the Internet that helps you find information on topics of interest, such as Yahoo and Google.

Emotional and Social Concerns

213

American Cancer Society (ACS)
Provides extensive information to patients and families on specific cancer types and treatments and on coping with cancer.
Internet: www.cancer.org
Telephone: 800-ACS-2345

Association of Cancer Online Resources
Provides information and support to cancer patients and to those who care for them through the creation and maintenance of cancer-related Internet mailing lists and Web-based resources.
Internet: www.acor.org

CancerCare
Provides free, professional support services to anyone affected by cancer: counseling and support groups, education, financial assistance, and practical help.
Internet: www.cancercare.org
Telephone: 800-813-HOPE (4673)

Cancer Information Network
Provides links to other Internet sites on specific types of cancers.
Internet: www.thecancer.info

Cancer Net
Developed by the American Society of Clinical Oncology, provides oncologist-approved cancer information.
Internet: www.cancer.net

Cancer Survivors Network
Sponsored by the American Cancer Society, provides a forum for communicating with other cancer survivors and has a listing of resources.
Internet: csn.cancer.org

CancerSymptoms.org
Developed by the Oncology Nursing Society, provides information
on managing commonly experienced treatment-related symptoms.
Internet: www.cancersymptoms.org

Lance Armstrong Foundation
The mission of this organization is to inspire and empower people
affected by cancer.
Internet: www.livestrong.org

National Cancer Institute (NCI)
Provides extensive information to patients and families on specific
cancer types and treatments and on coping with cancer.
Internet: www.cancer.gov
Telephone: 800-4-CANCER (Cancer Information Service)

National Coalition for Cancer Survivorship
A survivor-led cancer advocacy organization, with an additional
focus on patient education. The Cancer Survival Toolbox is a par-
ticularly valuable resource.
Internet: www.canceradvocacy.org
Telephone: 877-NCCS-YES

National Comprehensive Cancer Network (NCCN)
The consumer website of the NCCN, an alliance of leading cancer
centers dedicated to improving the quality and effectiveness of
care provided to cancer patients; clinical practice guidelines out-
line treatment recommendations for many cancers and cancer-
related side effects; provides information on living with cancer.
Internet: www.nccn.org

Oncolink
Sponsored by the University of Pennsylvania. The Coping section
addresses symptoms and side effects.
Internet: www.oncolink.com

Glossary

Acupuncture: a technique of inserting thin needles into the body at specific locations with the goal of restoring the normal flow of energy in the body; often used to treat pain or other symptoms.

Addiction: a desire or craving for the medication to feel high rather than to have your pain relieved.

Adjuvant chemotherapy: chemotherapy treatment used after a tumor has been removed surgically to destroy any remaining microscopic cancer cells (those that are unable to be seen with the naked eye) possibly left behind after surgery.

Advance directives: legal documents in which you indicate who you want to make medical decisions for you and/or what type of medical care you want to receive if you become unable to make decisions or speak for yourself in the future.

Analgesics: medications for treating pain.

Anemia: a low red blood cell count.

Antiemetics: medication used to prevent or treat nausea and vomiting.

Antihistamine: medication that is used to prevent or treat allergic reactions and that is sometimes given to treat itching caused by a rash.

Ascites: the abnormal buildup of fluid in the abdominal cavity.

Benign: noncancerous.

Biologic therapy: treatment with immune substances that destroy cancer cells or strengthen the ability of the immune system to destroy the cancer cells.

Botanicals: plants or plant parts valued for their medicinal properties; includes herbal products; commonly prepared as a tea, an extract, or a tincture.

Brachytherapy: radiation treatment that involves the placement of a sealed radioactive source (for example, a seed, wire, ribbon, or tube) into the body that emits radiation into the immediately surrounding area as it decays (or breaks down); also called implant or internal radiation.

Catheter: a thin flexible tube that is used to administer fluid into the body or to drain fluid from the body.

Cerebral edema: a swelling of the brain from inflammation or other diseases.

Chemotherapy: treatment with drugs that destroy cancer cells or stop them from growing.

Clinical trials: research studies to test the effectiveness of new treatments on humans.

Coagulation profile: a blood test that analyzes the clotting ability of the blood.

Cognitive dysfunction: difficulty remembering names, places, or events or trouble with language skills, concentration, or arithmetic.

Combined modality therapy: the use of a combination of treatments to destroy cancer cells.

Complete blood count (CBC): a blood test to measure the number of white blood cells, red blood cells, and platelets.

Computed tomography (CT): a diagnostic test that creates images of structures in the body using x-rays and a computer; slices or cuts of the body in a particular area can be seen.

Consent form: a written document signed by patients to indicate that they have been informed about a treatment, as well as the associated risks and benefits, and that they agree

to receive the treatment; also referred to as *informed consent.*

Cystitis: inflammation or irritation of the bladder.

Diuretic: a medication that increases the production of urine; also called a "water pill."

Do not resuscitate (DNR) order: an indication in a patient's medical chart based on the expressed wishes of the patient or their health care agent that no extraordinary life-extending measures are to be taken if they stop breathing or if their heart stops beating.

Doppler ultrasound: a procedure in which high-energy sound waves (ultrasound) are bounced off internal tissues or organs and make echoes that form a picture of body tissues, called a *sonogram;* can be used to determine whether there is a clot in a blood vessel in an arm or leg.

Dosimetrist: a member of the radiation oncology team who designs treatment plans and calculates the dose of radiation the tissues will receive when treated with radiation therapy; works in collaboration with a medical physicist and a radiation oncologist.

Dyspareunia: pain or discomfort during sexual intercourse.

Dyspnea: difficult or labored breathing; shortness of breath.

Dysuria: pain or burning on urination; usually caused by irritation or infection of the bladder or urethra (tube that empties the bladder).

Electrolytes: chemicals (e.g., sodium, potassium, chloride, and calcium) in the blood that help regulate nerve and muscle function and help the body maintain its balance of fluid.

Eligibility criteria: a list of conditions that must be met for someone to enroll in a clinical trial.

Emboli: blood clots that travel through blood vessels and that can obstruct or block the flow of blood.

Endocrinologist: a doctor who specializes in diagnosing and treating hormone disorders, including diabetes.

Endometriosis: a benign condition in which tissue similar to that which lines the uterus grows in abnormal places in the abdomen.

Extravasation: a potential complication of intravenous chemotherapy administration that occurs when chemotherapy leaks from the vein into the surrounding tissue.

Feeding tube: a tube placed through the nose or through the abdominal wall into the stomach to give liquid nutritional supplements.

Fluid retention: a condition in which the body does not eliminate adequate fluid and can cause swelling and weight gain.

Glucose: a type of sugar and the chief source of energy for living organisms.

Grade: a measure of how abnormal a cell appears when examined under a microscope; in some cases predicts how aggressive the cancer is.

Guided imagery: a technique in which patients use their imagination to visualize something they desire, such as visualizing the chemotherapy attacking their cancer cells.

Health care agent: a person designated to make health care decisions for you if you are not able to.

Hematocrit: the percentage of red cells in the blood.

Hemoglobin: the substance in red blood cells that binds to oxygen and carries it to the tissues of the body.

Hemoptysis: coughing up blood or blood-tinged sputum from the lower respiratory tract (below the throat) or lungs.

Homeopathic medicine: a treatment to stimulate the body's healing responses by giving extremely small doses of substances that produce symptoms of illness if given in larger doses.

Hormonal therapy: treatment that alters specific hormone levels in the body by stopping the production of the hormone, blocking the hormone, or adding hormone, thereby slowing or stopping the growth of the cancer cells.

Hospice: a program that provides supportive care to patients at the end of their life; can be provided at home or at an inpatient facility.

Hyperglycemia: abnormally high blood sugar.

Incontinence: the uncontrolled loss or leakage of urine.

Inferior vena cava filter: a filter (an umbrella-like device) that is placed in the inferior vena cava to prevent blood clots in the legs from traveling to the lungs.

Intensity-modulated radiation therapy: a method of planning and delivering radiation therapy that uses 3-dimensional images of the body to precisely aim multiple beams of radiation with varying intensities to the target tissue from many different angles; this minimizes the dose received by the surrounding normal tissues.

Internists: physicians who specialize in the diagnosis and medical treatment of adults.

Intraoperative radiation: the administration of radiation to the tumor site during surgery.

Jaundice: yellowing of the skin and the whites of the eyes resulting from a buildup of bilirubin in the tissues; it can occur if the bile ducts are blocked or if the liver is not functioning, and is accompanied by a darkening of the urine and a lightening of stool color.

Kegel exercises: exercises that are designed to increase muscle strength and elasticity in the pelvis and that may be recommended for treatment of urinary incontinence.

Linear accelerator: a machine that uses electricity to create high-energy radiation.

Lipids: fats.

Living will: a document in which you can state specific instructions regarding your health care, outlining which medical interventions you want to have performed and which you want to have withheld, given a variety of circumstances.

Locally advanced: a cancerous tumor has spread to surrounding structures.

Lymph nodes: bean-shaped structures in the lymphatic system that filter lymph fluid before it is returned to the bloodstream.

Lymphedema: a condition in which lymph fluid collects in tissues, usually in an arm or leg, after the removal or damage to lymph nodes from surgery or radiation therapy.

Macrobiotic diet: a diet that consists of whole grains and cereals that may be supplemented with beans and vegetables; varies in how restrictive it is and may not provide adequate nutrients.

Magnetic resonance imaging (MRI): a diagnostic test that creates images of structures in the body using radio waves and a powerful magnet.

Malignant: cancerous.

Metabolism: a series of chemical reactions in which cells convert nutrients to energy.

Metastasized: a cancerous tumor has spread to a distant site, such as the bones, the liver, or the brain.

Mucous membranes: thin tissues that line many of the cavities and passageways of the body, for example the gastrointestinal tract, the respiratory tract, and the genitourinary tract.

Myalgias: aches and pains in the muscles.

Naturopathic medicine: the use of a variety of "natural" therapies to enhance the body's healing forces.

Neoadjuvant chemotherapy: chemotherapy treatment given before the primary treatment (such as surgery) that is often used to shrink the tumor, making it easier for the surgeon to remove.

Nerve block: injecting a local anesthetic or alcohol into or around the nerve near the point where the tumor is pressing.

Nerve-sparing surgeries: surgical procedures for men with prostate cancer in which the prostate is surgically removed and the nerves are left undisturbed with the goal of maintaining erectile function.

Neurologist: a physician who takes care of people with problems or diseases of the nervous system.

Neutropenia: a decrease in the number of neutrophils, the type of white blood cell that fights bacterial infection and other diseases.

Neutrophils: a type of white blood cell that fights infection and other diseases.

Nocturia: frequent urination that occurs at night.

Obstruction: blockage in a passageway.

Oncologist: a physician who specializes in treating cancer; surgical oncologists specialize in cancer surgery; medical oncologists specialize in treatment with chemotherapy, hormonal therapy, and biologic therapy; radiation oncologists specialize in treating with radiation.

Oral mucositis: inflammation or irritation of the mucous membranes in the mouth; can be caused by chemotherapy or radiation therapy.

Osteoporosis: a condition characterized by a decrease in bone mass and density (thinning of the bones), causing bones to become fragile.

Palliation: treatment to relieve symptoms and to improve the quality of life.

Palliative care: a philosophy of care that helps patients achieve the best possible quality of life.

Paracentesis: a procedure in which a thin needle or tube is placed through the abdominal wall to remove fluid from the peritoneal cavity.

Paraneoplastic syndrome: a group of symptoms that may develop when substances released by some cancer cells disrupt the normal function of cells and tissue away from the tumor; it can be a cause of cognitive dysfunction.

Peripheral neuropathy: a condition of the nervous system that causes numbness, tingling, burning, or weakness; usually begins in the hands or feet and can be caused by certain anticancer drugs.

Peritoneal cavity: the space within the abdomen and pelvis that contains many structures, including the intestines and liver, and that is lined by thin membranes.

Platelets: cells in the blood that stop bleeding by clumping together, or clotting, to plug up damaged blood vessels; also called thrombocytes.

Pleural effusion: the abnormal buildup of fluid in the chest cavity.

Pleural space: the space between the membranes that line the inside of the

Glossary

chest wall and that cover the outside of the lungs.

Pleurodesis: a medical procedure that uses chemicals or drugs to cause inflammation and adhesion between the layers of the pleura to prevent the buildup of fluid in the pleural cavity.

Positron emission tomography (PET): a diagnostic test that creates images of the body based on metabolic activity; radioactive glucose (sugar) is injected, and because cancer cells have a higher metabolic rate than normal cells, the glucose will go to those cells and become visible on the scan.

Postherpetic neuralgia: localized pain that occurs in the area where shingles was present.

Prostate gland: a gland within the male reproductive system that is located just below the bladder surrounding part of the urethra, the canal that empties the bladder, and that produces a fluid that forms part of semen.

Prostatitis: inflammation or infection of the prostate gland in men.

Pruritus: a sensation that makes people want to scratch.

Psychiatric nurses: Registered nurses who care for patients with mental health issues; some provide counseling; nurse practitioners have advanced degrees and can prescribe medication.

Psychiatrists: doctors who specialize in the prevention, diagnosis, and treatment of mental illness; a psychiatrist can prescribe medicine.

Psychologists: specialists who can talk with patients and their families about emotional and personal matters and who can help them make decisions.

Pulmonary embolism: a blood clot in the lung; usually starts when a blood clot travels from a vein in the legs to the pulmonary artery, causing sudden shortness of breath.

Radiation therapy: the use of high-energy radiation to destroy cancer cells; also called radiotherapy.

Radioactive isotopes: unstable elements that emit radioactivity as they decay (break down); used to take diagnostic images or to treat cancer.

Radionuclide scanning: a diagnostic test that creates images of the body; after radioactive material is injected or swallowed, it collects in particular organs of the body; a scanner creates an image based on measurements of radioactivity in the organ.

Red blood cells: cells in the blood that contain hemoglobin that carries oxygen from the lungs to all the tissues in the body, which the cells use to create energy; also called erythrocytes.

Reiki: a technique of placing hands lightly on the body or just above it to facilitate the body's own healing responses.

Remission: a disappearance of all signs and symptoms of cancer.

Search engine: a service on the Internet that helps you find information on topics of interest, such as Yahoo and Google.

Shunt: allows fluid to move from one part of the body to another.

Social workers: professionals who are trained to talk with people and their families about emotional or physical needs and to find them support services.

Stage: a measure of how extensive the cancer is, that is, how much it has spread.

Stereotactic radiosurgery: a method of delivering multiple precisely defined beams of radiation to a small area of the brain in a single treatment.

Steroids: medications that are used to relieve inflammation and, in people with cancer, to prevent allergic reactions from chemotherapy and to ease other problems, such as nausea and vomiting, pain, shortness of breath, and loss of energy.

Thoracentesis: removal of fluid from the pleural cavity through a needle inserted between the ribs.

Three-dimensional conformal radiation therapy: a method of planning and delivering radiation therapy that uses 3-dimensional images of the body to precisely aim multiple beams of radiation to the target tissue from different angles; this minimizes the dose received by the surrounding normal tissues.

Thrombosis: the formation or presence of a blood clot inside a blood vessel.

Topical anesthetic: a medication applied to the surface of the body (for example, the skin or mucous membranes) to numb the area.

Tumor: an abnormal swelling or mass in the body.

Urologist: a specialist in problems or diseases of the urinary tract.

Vesicant: a type of chemotherapy that causes blistering or other local tissue damage if it leaks from a vein into the surrounding tissue.

White blood cells: cells in the blood that fight off infection and other types of disease; there are many different types of white blood cells, including neutrophils and lymphocytes; also called leukocytes.

Index

Chills, 57, 75, 120, 122, 163, 176
Chinese medicine, 23
Chiropractors, 23
Chronic pain, 51, 52, 63
Cialis, 145
Cigarette smoking, 182–184
Cimetidine, 110
Ciprofloxacin, 149
Cisplatin, 81, 84, 101, 128, 149
Clinical trials, 18–22
    consent form, 21
    costs of, 22, 41
    eligibility criteria, 21
    finding, 34–35, 41
    phases of, 20–21
Coagulation profile, 96, 160
Codeine, 50, 96
Cognitive dysfunction, 155–156, 171
Colace, 54
Cold sensitivity, 150
Colon cancer, 68
Colostomy, 6
Combined modality therapy, 5
Comfort measures. *See specific comfort measures*
Communication with doctor, 27–28, 32–34
Compazine (prochlorperazine), 114
Complementary and alternative
        medicine (CAM)
    deciding to use, 37–38
    descriptions of, 22–24
    emotional concerns, 189
    finding, 35–36
    for hot flashes, 137
    for itching, 61
    for menopause, 134–135, 137
    for nausea and vomiting, 111–112
    for pain management, 57
Complete blood count (CBC), 12, 67,
        72–73, 96, 170
Completion of treatment, 28–30, 193–195
Comprehensive cancer centers, 41
Compression stockings, 158
Computed tomography (CT)
    ascites, 164
    cerebral edema, 152
    during chemotherapy, 11
    contrast material, side effects, 81
    evaluation of treatment, 27, 28
    hemoptysis, evaluation of, 96
    lymphedema, 163
    radiation therapy, 7
    stage of tumor, determination of, 2
Concentration, problems with, 134, 155,
        192, 218

Conception after treatment, 140–143
Confusion and memory changes, 55,
        155–156, 171
Congestive heart failure, 92
Consent form for clinical trials, 21
Constipation, 3, 55, 116–118
Coping with diagnosis, 186–189
    decision making on treatment, 40–43
    information on illness and prognosis,
        27–28
    recurrence or spread of cancer, treatment
        goals, 27–28
Coronary heart disease. *See* Heart disease
Corticosteroids. *See* Steroids
Costs
    of clinical trials, 22, 41
    of prescription medications, 211
    tax deduction for, 211–212
Coughing
    blood from, 95–96
    as cancer symptom, 3, 4
    infections and, 75
Coumadin (warfarin), 160–161
Coworkers and work, 198–201
Creams, for itching, 61
Creative therapies, 23
Crushing medication, 105–106
CT. *See* Computed tomography
Cure, defined, 28
Curél, 61
CyberKnife systems, 7
Cyclophosphamide, 101, 119, 121, 122
Cystitis, 119, 121
Cytokines, 15

D

Dacarbazine, 58
Darbepoetin (Aranesp), 64, 67, 68, 76, 156
Decadron (dexamethasone), 81, 114, 128, 153
Decision making
    advance directives, 44–47
    on treatment, 40–43
Deep vein thrombosis (DVT), 157,
        158–161
Dehydration, 171
Dental work, preparation for, 180
Dentures, adjustment of, 103
Depression. *See* Emotional and social concerns
Dexamethasone (Decadron), 81, 114,
        128, 153
Diabetes, 106, 117, 120, 154, 171–173,
        180, 181
Diagnosis
    coping with. *See* Coping with diagnosis

Index